The International Library of Sociology

MENTAL HOSPITALS AT WORK

Founded by KARL MANNHEIM

The International Library of Sociology

THE SOCIOLOGY OF MENTAL HEALTH

In 7 Volumes

MENTAL HOSPITALS AT WORK

by

KATHLEEN JONES

and

ROY SIDEBOTHAM

Routledge
Taylor & Francis Group
LONDON AND NEW YORK

First published in 1962 by
Routledge and Kegan Paul Ltd

Reprinted in 1998 by
Routledge
2 Park Square, Milton Park,
Abingdon, Oxon, OX14 4RN

Simultaneously published in the USA and Canada by Routledge
711 Third Avenue, New York, NY 10017

Transferred to digital print 2013

Routledge is an imprint of the Taylor & Francis Group, an informa business

First issued in paperback 2013

© 1962 Kathleen Jones and Roy Sidebotham

All rights reserved. No part of this book may be reprinted or reproduced or utilized in any form or by any electronic, mechanical, or other means, now known or hereafter invented, including photocopying and recording, or in any information storage or retrieval system, without permission in writing from the publishers.

The publishers have made every effort to contact authors/copyright holders of the works reprinted in *The International Library of Sociology*. This has not been possible in every case, however, and we would welcome correspondence from those individuals/companies we have been unable to trace.

British Library Cataloguing in Publication Data
A CIP catalogue record for this book
is available from the British Library

Mental Hospitals at Work

ISBN 978-0-415-17805-1 (hbk)
ISBN 978-0-415-86418-3 (pbk)

CONTENTS

TABLES

(All tables refer to Crown Lodge, Northtown and Moordale, and to the year 1957–8 unless otherwise stated)

TABLES

PREFACE

This study was made possible by a grant from the Nuffield Provincial Hospitals Trust. We acknowledge our debt to the Trustees, and our gratitude to their secretary, Mr. Gordon McLachlan, for his help and encouragement.

The idea for the research originated with Dr. W. V. Wadsworth, medical superintendent of Cheadle Royal. Dr. Wadsworth has kept in touch throughout the research period, and has contributed much from his own experience to our understanding of psychiatric administration. Dr. W. L. Tonge, consultant psychiatrist to the United Sheffield Hospitals, also gave valuable advice. Mrs. Heather Price, formerly social worker to the Townleys branch of Bolton General Hospital, acted as research assistant. This was essentially an interdisciplinary project, and we should like to record our gratitude to all three for the contributions which they have made in discussion from their own professional viewpoints.

The following have been kind enough to read the completed manuscript, and to make suggestions for improvement: Professor T. E. Chester, Mr. Arthur Blenkinsop, Mr. C. Montacute and Mrs. B. N. Rodgers, of the University of Manchester, and Professor G. R. Hargreaves, of the University of Leeds. Though they are in no way responsible for our conclusions, and any inaccuracies remain our own responsibility, we are most grateful for their advice and help.

The medical superintendents and staff of the hospitals which we studied in detail cannot unfortunately be mentioned by name, as we have used pseudonyms throughout to ensure greater freedom of comment. They endured our questioning and observation with much courtesy and patience, and their friendly assistance turned what might have been an invidious task into a very pleasant one. In all three hospitals we were free to make whatever enquiries we wished, without reservations of any kind.

Thanks are also due to the workers in the community services

—general practitioners, psychiatric social workers, mental welfare officers, and others—who provided material for the follow-up study, often at some personal inconvenience; and to Miss Rosemary Churchill, Miss Valerie Cleaver, Miss Pauline Hickson, Mr. Paul Taylor, and Mr. Ronald Walton, formerly students and now graduates of the University of Manchester, who worked as assistant nurses in the three hospitals, and provided corroborative material on nursing problems and patient-groupings. Miss Mary Stewart and Miss Jean Stewart were responsible for deciphering, typing and checking the manuscript, and we should like to thank them also.

It is not possible to do 'consumer research' in mental hospitals, for although patients often have very decided views, these are frequently conditioned by their illness and their own subjective experiences. Nevertheless, it is important that the patients' own viewpoint should not be lost among a welter of administrative and statistical considerations, and we were fortunate in that a number of patients, meeting us on the wards and in the corridors, took a considerable interest in the project. They contributed observations and anecdotes from their own experience, and these were carefully checked by reference to medical or nursing staff, or to records. We are grateful to these patients—many of whom are now back in their own homes, and living normal lives at the time of writing—for a constant reminder of the human values which underlie this or any other piece of research into mental illness.

K. J.
R. S.

The University of Manchester, 1961.

INTRODUCTION

In recent years, statistics have shown a considerable change in the role of the mental hospital within the Mental Health Services.

From 1842, when official statistics were first collected by the Metropolitan Commissioners in Lunacy, a regular yearly rise in the number of patients resident in mental hospitals was noted. This continued steadily until 1954, the only exceptions being in the war years, when facilities for treatment were severely limited. Small mental hospitals were extended. Counties which had initially built one found themselves obliged to build two or three or more. Even so, there were never enough beds to meet the demand, and a chronic shortage of accommodation was accepted as a permanent feature in the situation.

In 1954–5, this long-standing trend was abruptly reversed. The figures for 1955 showed the first peace-time decrease in resident populations, of 1,288. Subsequent years have shown further decreases, each year's total being lower than that of the year before. In all, between 1954 and 1959, official statistics for patients resident in mental hospitals showed a drop of over 16,000.

A rising curve has thus been replaced, for these few years, by a falling curve; and there is a good deal of discussion as to what this means. In some quarters, it is believed that the decline will continue irresistibly and of its own momentum until the mental hospitals are empty. In others, that while the continuation of this trend is not inevitable, it is desirable in view of the unsatisfactory service offered by mental hospitals; and that it should be hastened by the provision of extended community services and psychiatric beds in general hospitals.

We do not subscribe to either of these views. While we welcome the extension of community services, which is long overdue in some areas, we believe that the mental hospital still has an important part to play in the Mental Health Services, and that it is unwise either to accelerate the pace of change or to exaggerate its scope.

If 'the decline of the mental hospital' is exaggerated in official and professional pronouncements, the tentative attempts which have been made since 1948 to close the gap in standards between mental hospitals and other hospitals will come to an end. Ambitious and progressively-minded staff will leave the mental hospital for other forms of employment. Research and clinical advance may be slowed for lack of facilities. Mental hospitals will face a decline in their resources of men and money and talent at a time when these resources, always meagre, are needed more than ever before. It is in the belief that this would be a serious loss to the Mental Health Services as a whole that this book is presented.

This is a study of what mental hospitals actually do, what problems they face, how they use their resources, and how their efficiency can be assessed. We begin in Part I by briefly describing the provision of mental hospitals in England and Wales, and analysing current trends in hospital and community care, together with the arguments for and against the retention of the mental hospital.

Part II consists of a detailed study of three hospitals at work. There are many factors which cannot be adequately evaluated in a generalized way at national level, and which require specific detail for their elucidation. We have therefore described and analysed the work of three very different hospitals—a small private hospital where the standard fee is 15 guineas a week and the 'therapeutic community' system is practised; a large Health Service hospital, formerly a county asylum; and a small Health Service hospital with some amenity and private beds, which is associated with a university Department of Psychiatry. These hospitals, each of which is situated in a different Regional Hospital Board area, were chosen for their potentialities of contrast.

The account of their work is largely written in the present tense for ease of reading, but it refers in fact to a limited period of time—June 1958 to June 1959. The pattern has been caught and preserved in a series of case-studies; but there have been administrative and clinical changes in all three since June 1959, and it would be unfair if this analysis should be taken to refer to them at the date of publication, or at some later date of reading.

The names of the hospitals and of individuals connected with them have been altered, to prevent exact identification, and to allow a greater freedom of comment. Minor details in some of the incidents recorded have been changed for the same reason. With these exceptions, all recorded material is authentic.

In Part III, we use statistics from the three hospitals as illustrative material in considering indices of efficiency. Judgements on what constitutes a 'good' hospital or a 'bad' hospital are often made on a very superficial basis. One hospital will be praised because its buildings are modern, and another condemned because they are old. Professor Parkinson has some interesting views on this subject.[1] A hospital may become known as 'the one with a good rehabilitation policy' or 'the one where Dr. X. did that paper on schizophrenia', and such casually-applied tags will stick long after the rehabilitation scheme has died of inanition, or Dr. X. has accepted a fellowship in America.

There are, of course, more adequate criteria of judgement. Qualitative assessments are constantly being made by a variety of visitors, from Ministry officials to patients' relatives. Commissioners of the old Board of Control developed an almost psychic power of evaluation in their routine visitations. There have also been many attempts to estimate efficiency in quantitative terms, from the early nineteenth-century rating of 'cures' to the more sophisticated modern devices of follow-up studies and cost accounting. We come to the conclusion that no simple measure of efficiency is adequate, and after considering several suggestions for complex measures, make a suggestion of our own in terms of 'cost per case'.

Part IV consists of some general observations on organizational problems, and conclusions about the future needs and potentialities of mental hospitals.

Throughout, 'mental hospital' has been used in preference to the newer usage of 'psychiatric hospital' since the latter term also includes mental deficiency hospitals, which are not within the scope of this survey.

[1] *Parkinson's Law*, pp. 84–5: 'A perfection of planned lay-out is only achieved by institutions on the point of collapse . . . during the period of exciting discovery or progress, there is no time to plan the perfect headquarters.'

PART ONE

The Mental Hospital Today

I

THE IMPACT OF CHANGE

At the time of writing, there are about 130 hospitals in England and Wales which are separately administered, and which receive mental patients exclusively, or almost exclusively. Of these, two have more than 3,000 beds each;[1] 22 have between 2,000 and 3,000 beds; 48 have between 1,000 and 2,000 beds; 30 have between 500 and 1,000 beds; and the rest have less than 500 beds.

Large mental hospitals occur in two main concentrations: on the fringes of the Greater London area, and in a belt across the Liverpool, Manchester and Leeds conurbations. Small hospitals are generally in less populous areas, such as Somerset, Gloucestershire, or Suffolk.

Most mental hospitals operating today were constructed between 1850 and 1914. There seem to have been two main waves of building, following the Lunatics Act of 1845 and the Lunacy Act of 1890. Only two mental hospitals of more than 1,000 beds have been set up since the First World War.

The Mental Treatment Act of 1930 introduced provision for voluntary patients, and most mental hospital committees made special provision by means of new 'admission units' or 'neurosis units' for the milder types of cases then admitted.

In addition to these hospitals administered by Regional Hospital Boards, there is one post-graduate teaching hospital group, Bethlem and the Maudsley, and there are four 'registered hospitals'.

[1] It is normal practice to refer to patient numbers in terms of 'beds'. In fact, of course, most patients are ambulant.

The Bethlem-Maudsley group is a unique combination of the old and the new. Bethlem, the oldest mental hospital in England, originated in a monastic foundation of 1272, and, after a somewhat chequered history, was rebuilt on a new site in 1930. The Maudsley, built immediately before the First World War, was not opened to civilian patients until 1923, when it fulfilled its benefactor's intention by becoming the first mental hospital to take early, recoverable cases without certificate.[1] The two hospitals were administratively united in 1948, and the group is directly responsible to the Ministry of Health.

The four registered hospitals are private, non-profit-making hospitals with a recognized standing. At present, they have about 1,200 beds between them.

In addition, there are increasing numbers of annexes and wings of general hospitals which make provision for psychiatric patients, but are not separately administered, and numbers of small mental nursing homes, which are now inspected by the local authority. These establishments are not included in this survey.

The detailed figures for resident populations and admissions to mental hospitals in the years 1952–9 are as follows:

TABLE 1

Admissions and Resident Populations of Mental Hospitals in England and Wales, 1952–9*

	Total admitted	Total resident Dec. 31st	+ or − on total resident in previous year
1952	68,619	149,353	
1953	73,493	151,378	+2,025
1954	78,583	152,144	+ 766
1955	83,392	150,856	−1,288
1956	89,323	149,480	−1,376
1957	94,020	146,962	−2,518
1958		141,628	−5,334
1959	98,237	136,138	−5,490

* From *Annual Reports of the Ministry of Health*, H.M.S.O. No figure for admissions was published in the Report for 1958.

[1] By means of a special Act of Parliament. This was prior to the Mental Treatment Act.

It will be seen that the increase in resident populations was already slowing up in 1954. In 1955, it changed to a decrease for the first time, and the yearly decrease has since been progressively larger.

The reasons for this change are complex. To some extent, advances in clinical psychiatry seem to be responsible—in particular, the introduction of new ranges of drugs since 1954. The 'open-door policy'—a term which includes not only the use of unlocked wards, but also new kinds of therapeutic activity, and the development of part-time treatment[1]—was introduced concurrently. The Mental Health Act introduced informal admission and discharge for the first time, but some hospital authorities had anticipated this by admitting patients informally to 'de-designated' wards. There is a major change in policy—the belief that patients should in most cases only enter hospital during the acute phase or phases of their illness, and that several short periods of hospitalization are preferable to one long one. This has led to the open-door policy being nicknamed 'the revolving door policy', since one patient may enter hospital half a dozen times in the course of a year.

Alternative methods of care are developing, though it is doubtful whether they yet have an appreciable effect on in-patient statistics. Psychiatric units attached to general hospitals are one form of alternative. In the Manchester Region, a policy of providing peripheral units of this type for the city population has been officially adopted, and other regions have initiated similar though less ambitious schemes. There is a growth in community care. Local authority Mental Health Departments were set up in 1948 with theoretically almost unlimited powers under section 28 of the National Health Service Act. The Mental Health Act 1959 defined some of these powers, particularly with regard to the provision of residential services, such as hostels and 'half-way houses', and local authorities were then required to submit schemes to the Minister of Health.

There are thus many factors at work simultaneously, and the situation has well been named one of 'therapeutic flux'. As a result, a number of forecasts have been made of the immediate

[1] i.e. day treatment, night treatment, week-day treatment, week-end treatment, and so on.

decline and ultimate abolition of the mental hospital. The Minister of Health stated in March 1961 that he expected the acute populations of mental hospitals to drop by half in the next 15 years, and the long-stay populations ultimately to dwindle to zero.[1] Dr. Alan Norton, in a survey of patients admitted to a mental hospital over the last 30 years, has suggested that 'the decrease in the number of schizophrenic illnesses becoming chronic may well lead to a fall in the total population of 30 per cent over the next 20 years. If, in addition, changes in national policy are effected, mental hospitals may perhaps be reduced to a quarter of their present size.'[2] Dr. A. A. Baker writes, 'Some people think that, with modern therapeutic advances, rehabilitation, and improved social services, a time will come when there are no long-stay patients,' and concludes, after an examination of patient statistics in his own hospital, 'If our present policies continue, and the community provides help in resettlement, I think that the hospital will continue to empty.'[3]

It will be seen that these forecasts involve three rather different types of argument: the clinical argument that illnesses formerly insusceptible to treatment are now being treated successfully, so that the prevalence of mental illness is being reduced; the statistical argument that, whatever the causes, a decline in the need for beds is in fact taking place, and is likely to continue; and the social argument that patients ought to be treated outside the mental hospital, and that we shall find ways of doing this successfully within the next few years. None of these arguments stands alone. Each is introduced to support the others.

Dr. G. C. Tooth of the Ministry of Health and Miss E. M. Brooke of the General Register Office, in a consideration of their statistical work in this field, comment: 'It seems unlikely that trends of this magnitude based on national figures are no more than temporary phenomena; though many factors may modify the rate of change, the direction seems to be well established'; but they also point out that there are 'trends which may have

[1] Inaugural speech to the Annual Conference of the National Association for Mental Health, 9th March 1961. Circular H.M. (61) 25 of 28th March.

[2] A. Norton, 'Mental Hospital Ins and Outs', *B.M.J.*, 25th February 1961.

[3] A. A. Baker, 'Pulling Down the Old Mental Hospital', *Lancet*, 25th March 1961.

the reverse effect'.[1] We now proceed to put the case for the mental hospital, and to discuss some of these trends.

1. *The actual decline in resident populations is smaller than it appears to be.* We have reproduced in Table 1 statistics which show a decline between 1954 and 1959 of over 16,000 beds. During this period, 9,312 beds were de-designated,[2] and these are not included in the later figures, though they were still in use. The real decline was thus not 16,000 but about 7,000—less than half.

2. *The existing beds are not yet even adequate to the need.* Despite this decline, there is still an excess of patients over authorized bed-space, amounting at 31st December 1959 to 7·6 per cent statutory overcrowding. The excess of patients over adequate and satisfactory accommodation is very much greater.

3. *The decline is unlikely to continue indefinitely of its own momentum.* There is no valid reason for assuming that numbers will continue to go down until they reach zero. After an up-curve which has continued for 112 years, it seems rash to project a similar down-curve on the basis of five or six years' evidence.

Recent improvements in clinical treatment are limited in their effects. The use of thymoleptics and other associated drugs has been valuable in the treatment of depression, but though the acute phase of an illness can now be treated more rapidly, this does not necessarily mean that it will not recur at a later date. The introduction of the phenothiazine derivatives has enabled some patients suffering from schizophrenia to remain in the community for a few years longer, but these drugs do not cure the disease entity known as schizophrenia. They may also be used to mitigate the symptoms of the senile psychoses, but again they do not affect the underlying pathological processes.

Short-stay patients often return for further periods of treatment in hospital—we give some figures later which indicate that, in the three hospitals surveyed, the relapse rate after one admission is about 30 per cent in the first two years.[3] Reduction in the numbers of long-stay patients over the past few years has been comparatively easy, because there were some stabilized patients who were quite capable of living in the community, given a little help; but unless a cure for schizophrenia is

[1] G. C. Tooth and E. M. Brooke, 'Trends in the Mental Hospital Population and their Effect on Future Planning', *Lancet*, 1st April 1961.

[2] Ibid.

[3] See p. 144, table 15.

discovered (and this could alter the whole situation) numbers really may well level off as we come to the hard core of patients who need hospital care.[1]

With the increase in longevity, we can expect the number of psychogeriatric patients to go up considerably, and this may balance the decrease in other directions.

4. *The growth in the community services is not likely to be adequate in the next few years to deal with a major reduction in the mental hospital population.* What are the facts about the community services as they operate today? Out-patient clinics have increased in numbers since 1948, but many offer only a minimal service, and appear to be mainly devices for keeping in touch with patients between breakdowns. Since psychiatrists often have to travel long distances to attend clinics, indefinite expansion is not possible without a considerable increase in the numbers of psychiatrists, and might well be uneconomic.

Local authority Mental Health Departments are, as the Younghusband Report has shown, seriously understaffed.[2] Few have a psychiatric social worker, and many of the staff employed are untrained, or at best partly trained. Though the proposals of the Younghusband Committee include a doubling of existing staff, this will involve competition with other avenues of work open to people of similar calibre, such as teaching and nursing, where recruitment problems are also severe. Many local authorities already have posts on their existing establishment which they are unable to fill. The creation of more unfilled posts, or the appointment of untrained people who undergo a merely nominal in-training, is not the answer.

This is difficult and exacting work. Not every social worker—or indeed every P.S.W.—is suited to it. The new training scheme for social workers suggested by the Younghusband Committee will, it is hoped, affect the situation favourably in time; but it would be unrealistic to expect these two-year trained workers to do the sustained case-work necessary without proper supervision, or to expect them to be forthcoming in adequate numbers unless standards are drastically dropped. As far as

[1] See C. P. Gore and K. Jones, Survey of a Long-stay Mental Hospital Population, *Lancet*, 2nd September 1961.

[2] Report of Working Party on Social Workers in the Local Authority Health and Welfare Services, H.M.S.O., 1959.

psychiatric social workers are concerned, Professor R. M. Titmuss has pointed out that, at the present rate of increase in numbers, it will take rather more than half a century for them to reach the Younghusband recommendations for local authority employment.[1]

How far are the new and extended proposals put up by the local authorities likely to be translated into fact? The answer to this question depends partly on the supply of workers, but partly also on financial policy. Since the introduction of the block grant in 1959, there has been no specific provision for the Mental Health Services of local authorities, and we have no guarantee that all local authorities will consider this a priority. There are so many entirely reasonable excuses which may be offered for failure to implement proposals—lack of money, inability to obtain building sites, lack of staff—that development may well be slow and will certainly be uneven.

Day hospitals have received a good deal of publicity, but the movement is smaller than is generally supposed. To date, there are only 50 or 60 in operation, and some of these are very small. The total number of patients attending is not much in excess of 1,500, and many of these patients attend for only one or two days a week.[2]

Although a day hospital is cheaper to build than a full mental hospital, since it requires no dormitory accommodation, the saving on capital costs may be offset by increased maintenance costs. Transport costs are negligible in centres of dense population, but can be high in rural or suburban areas. Some social workers consider that day hospitals require a higher social work staffing than in-patient hospitals, since the patient has constantly to adapt to two different environments, and the home situation needs careful consideration. Since in most cases the local authority provides both transport and social workers, these are concealed costs in that they do not appear in the day hospital's accounts; but they must be taken into consideration, and we cannot expect the day hospital movement to extend indefinitely outside populous areas.

[1] Address to the Annual Conference of the National Association for Mental Health, 10th March 1961.

[2] W. A. J. Farndale, *The Day Hospital Movement in Great Britain*, Pergamon Press, 1961.

Day attendances are suitable for patients with a good home environment, enabling them to keep in touch with their normal background rather than entering hospital and then having to go through a process of rehabilitation. They are not suitable for patients with difficult home environments and unsympathetic relatives, and it may be that the daily adaptation to two environments lengthens the course of treatment in some cases.

It is difficult to comment on hostels, since very few are yet in operation; but one can foresee the usual difficulties in finding sites (Tenants' Associations often raise objections to having such neighbours, on the grounds that their presence 'lowers the neighbourhood', upsets the children, and reduces the value of their property). Money and staff may also be hard to find. It is important that hostels should be pleasant, well-equipped places, and not workhouses under another name; that they should take only patients who really do not require the full facilities of a mental hospital; and that those for long-stay patients should accommodate well-matched and sociable groups, not a miscellaneous assortment of mental cripples. If all these factors are taken into consideration, the rather wild claim, sometimes heard at psychiatric meetings, that 'we shall soon close the mental hospitals and put all the patients in hostels' is seen to be distinctly over-optimistic.

This is perhaps a gloomy view of the community services. One would not wish to detract from the excellent work which is being done, and the energy, patience and integrity of the people who do it. The pity of it is that there are so few of them; that they often have to work under unsuitable conditions, without secretarial help, dependent on public transport for domiciliary visiting, and desperately conscious of how little can really be achieved under present circumstances.

In urban areas, it may be possible to introduce an adequate community service for patients of good home background in time. It will never be possible to provide a service which can deal with patients from difficult homes, except by taking them into hostel or hospital. It may prove that in many cases the mental hospital is the more satisfactory alternative.

5. *The development of psychiatric units in general hospitals provides a valuable means of treating some patients, but is unsuitable for the majority.* To some extent, terminology beclouds the issue here.

We have replaced the specific terminology of an earlier age—'lunatics', 'asylums', 'attendants', with terms borrowed from the general hospital—'patients', 'hospitals' and 'nurses'. Thus we may use the same terms as the general hospital in describing very different things.

Few general hospitals have adequate provision for ambulant patients. If they are allowed up, they must sit by their beds in dressing-gowns, or walk about the ward. The major part of the hospital consists of wards in which they are nursed, not of a community in which they live. The architecture and layout of a mental hospital, on the other hand, usually reflect the fact that most patients are mobile. A 'ward' is not a single room containing rows of beds, but a complex of rooms for different purposes. There are rooms for specific activities outside the ward—a hall for dances and meetings, a shop, a canteen, a library. There is space in the grounds for outdoor activities—walking, cricket, football, tennis, and sometimes gardening.

A mental hospital is basically planned for patient activity, and therefore requires space. Most mental hospitals were built in the country, partly because public prejudice drove them out of the towns, but partly also because rural land is cheaper than urban land, and they required a great deal of it. Though a general hospital can perfectly well be built upwards in the heart of a city, a mental hospital needs to spread outwards. If a psychiatric unit is attached to a general hospital, or existing wards are converted to psychiatric use, these factors are seldom taken into consideration.

Mental nursing has a different orientation from general nursing. The aim of the good general nurse is to care for her patient, and the patient's role is necessarily a dependent one. The aim of the good psychiatric nurse is to foster the patient's independence, to co-operate with him until he is capable of making his own decisions. Talking to patients, taking an interest in their emotional reactions and hopes for the future, are more important than the ritual of pulse- and temperature-taking. The stringent discipline and order which may be necessary in the acute general hospital are quite out of place in dealing with psychiatric patients, who need a slower pace and a more personal relationship with the nursing staff. Yet in fact, most psychiatric patients in general hospitals are nursed by general nurses; and even where psychiatrically-trained nurses are employed, they come under the direction of the general nursing hierarchy.

There are some advantages in sending mental patients to general hospitals—the lack of stigma in treatment, and the fact that visiting is easier for patients in a town centre. The disadvantages may not matter for a patient who is only to remain in hospital for a week or two, and for patients suffering from the known psychosomatic disorders, general hospital treatment may be definitely indicated; but it is a poor service to the average patient if, in order to avoid a now largely illusory stigma, we deny him the special conditions which only the mental hospital can adequately provide. Integration of general and psychological medical services at the national and regional level was achieved in 1948, with subsequent benefit to both. It is logical, but not sensible, to pursue integration at the clinical level.

6. *A family-centred service must be prepared to admit patients to hospital on social as well as medical criteria.* There is a tendency to talk of patients 'needing' treatment on purely clinical grounds, and estimates of the demand for beds in general hospitals are usually based on the concept of clinical need.[1] In the case of mental illness, the need is often a social one, since the symptoms are behavioural. Some patients find the home atmosphere too stressful during the period of treatment, particularly if there are marital or other problems in human relationships. Twenty-three hours with a nagging wife can undo the good done in one hour with a psychiatrist. Though from a strictly clinical point of view the treatment could be given in a day hospital or an out-patient clinic, it is not likely to be successful while the patient remains in an emotionally-charged environment. Though the word 'asylum' has now become tainted with unhappy associations, there is sound sense in the idea of a refuge from the cares of the world, a temporary, sheltered environment for treatment.

There are other cases where it might indeed be beneficial for the patient if he could stay at home but where this would place an unwarrantable stress on the rest of the family circle. For example, some child psychiatrists are already deeply concerned

[1] See R. Logan and G. Forsyth, *The Demand for Medical Care*, Nuffield/O.U.P., 1960.

about the effect on young children of the presence in the family circle of confused and deluded grandparents. It is easy to say 'The family must bear the burden', but every social worker knows families where the burden is not just one, but two or three difficult members, and it is only borne at the cost of tremendous physical and mental strain. If we think in terms of positive mental health (and not just of reducing the bills for mental illness in the next few years) we must consider the needs of the whole family, and the health of all its members.

This question raises deep and often insoluble problems in human priorities; but the right answer is not always and inevitably 'The family must cope'.

7. *Public tolerance of mental disorder has increased in the last few years, but may decrease again.* We cannot assume a growing tolerance, particularly where the more seriously disordered patients are concerned. While most mental patients require only a little sympathy and understanding, there are still some who are capable of anti-social acts. It is too early to say yet whether there is a correlation between the policy of early discharge and the apparent rise in crimes of violence and sex offences;[1] but if such a correlation should be proved—or even thought to exist—public tolerance could decline very sharply. A Press and television campaign could kill the open-door policy almost overnight. While every effort must be made to stop this from happening, we must realize that a too-hasty policy of discharging patients could in itself be the precipitating factor.

In this connection, it is interesting to note that the Dutch authorities, who have carried out pioneer work in the development of parole and community care, in 1961 requested psychiatrists to exercise greater caution in this respect.[2] If public tolerance is to be maintained in this country, it is important that we should not try it too severely, and that we should proceed with care in releasing those whose actions might constitute a danger or an offence to the ordinary citizen.

8. *Full employment reduces the mental hospital population: trade*

[1] Dr. T. Morris and L. Blom-Cooper ('An Analysis of Murder', *The Observer*, 16th April 1961) suggest that the proportion of known or suspected killers suffering from mental disorder since the passing of the Homicide Act 1957 is about 65 per cent; but a great deal depends upon definition, and it is difficult to get comparable earlier figures.

[2] *The Guardian*, 30th November 1960.

recessions increase it. The considerable rise in the demand for mental hospital beds in the nineteen-thirties was due not only to the effects of the Mental Treatment Act, but also to widespread unemployment. During a time of full employment, as at present, people with quite acute psychological problems are often able to find work and to maintain their maximum, though very limited, efficiency. When work becomes scarce, they are the first to be dismissed, and their mental condition is such that they cannot deal with the additional problems, financial and often emotional, resulting from dismissal. A policy of community care is thus very dependent on economic prosperity. If a trade recession should come, we should be faced with a larger demand for mental hospital beds at a time when we had not the resources to provide them.

9. *Past experience shows that new provisions reveal new demands.* As each type of psychiatric provision has come into being, it has brought an additional demand for treatment, rather than relieving pressure on existing agencies. This is a common experience in many types of social provision, for while human resources are limited, human needs are seemingly endless. Out-patient clinics did not reduce the demand for in-patient beds, even in the more prosperous years of the late thirties. There is some evidence that day hospitals, which were expected to reduce the pressure on both in-patient beds and out-patient clinics, have done neither. Many day hospital patients are part of a separate group which would not otherwise receive treatment.[1] We have no idea how great the true psychiatric need in the community is, and no way of measuring it; but it is possible that psychiatric units in general hospitals and local authority hostels will be called upon to tackle problems which are at present almost unrecognized for lack of provision. There is no guarantee at all that they will reduce pressure on in-patient beds on a one-for-one basis.

10. *Mental hospitals are at present carrying a greater volume of work than at any time in their history.* Table I shows that a consideration of resident populations gives only a partial picture of what is happening to mental hospitals. There are two ways of measuring these populations: taking a count of patients resident at any one time—31st December is the official date for Ministry statis-

[1] W. A. J. Farndale, *The Day Hospital Movement in Great Britain.*

tics—gives a static view. The other way is to count the number of patients admitted in any one year—and this number has continued steadily to increase. In other words, mental hospitals are now dealing with more patients than ever before—but discharging them more quickly. They may need less beds in future; but since there is no sign of a drop in admissions, they will need more staff, more equipment, and more money.

11. *The demand for 'the decline of the mental hospital' springs largely from irrational and unacknowledged sources.* There are two very powerful motives behind the arguments against the mental hospital—one psychological, and the other financial.

First, mental hospitals are not popular, and the causes of this unpopularity lie deep in human personality. Admittedly, some mental hospitals have a grim past—though few of them were ever quite as bad as their detractors said they were.[1] Most of them have tackled an enormous task with chronic shortages of money and staff, and with very little public sympathy. They were not unpopular because they were bad; they were bad because they were unpopular.

Hostility and aggression spring from fear. Fear of being mentally ill, of losing one's rational judgement and independence of action, is so universal a human emotion that few of us escape it altogether, though we may disguise it in a number of ways. In an age which is too compassionate to release that fear, as earlier generations have done, in persecution of the mentally sick themselves, aggression tends to be switched to the therapist, or to the institution in which he works.

Laughter, Freud tells us, originates more often in fear and tension than in pure humour. In the eighteenth century, as is well known, young men about town amused themselves by baiting the lunatics in Bedlam. Today, when jokes about the mentally ill are no longer generally acceptable, jokes about psychiatrists and mental hospitals are still common.

Fear of the mental hospital leads to a desire to destroy it. This may be expressed in jokes about 'loony bins' and 'nuthouses'. It may also be expressed in a calm and superficially rational assumption that the mental hospital belongs to the

[1] This reference is to mental hospitals (county asylums) and not to the private madhouses of the early nineteenth century. Evidence shows that many of the latter were quite as bad as their detractors said they were.

unenlightened past, and that it is 'progressive' to look forward to its dissolution. There is more than one road to destruction.

If the fear motive is buried deep in the national subconscious, the financial motive is also generally unacknowledged. Mental hospitals, properly built and equipped, cost a good deal of money. Other types of psychiatric provision are initially cheaper to organize. They can be run on a shoe-string without this fact being readily apparent, for it is not easy to test the efficiency of the service which they offer.

Since 1948, the concept of the Health Service as a free and maximal service, providing for all the health needs of the population, has become somewhat tarnished. Probably it was an unattainable ideal, for as we have shown, human needs seem to be unlimited in this as in other respects; but successive governments have made energetic attempts to cut health expenditure, and in the mental health field the development of community care has provided a way of theoretically reconciling good service with lower costs. Thus it is frequently claimed that out-patient clinics are 'cheaper and better for the patient'. Hostels are 'cheaper and better for the patient'. Day hospitals are 'cheaper and better for the patient'. Some psychiatrists in day hospitals have claimed that it is therapeutically valuable for old age pensioners to pay for their midday meal. The phrase 'cheaper and better for the patient' has been repeated so often that it almost appears to be one proposition instead of two, though economy is no guarantee of better service.

There can be no doubt that the financial motive plays a considerable part in the move away from the mental hospital. It is cheaper for the Government of the day to find other methods of care than to repair the neglect and parsimony of the past and bring mental hospitals up to an acceptable standard. In the long run, this may not be the most economical policy.

12. *Dispersal of limited resources is ultimately more expensive and less efficient than concentration.* Psychiatrists, qualified mental nurses, and psychiatric social workers are in short supply, and likely to remain so. If we disperse available staff over many different types of organization, time is wasted, team-work is difficult, and the working day is fragmented. For example, a psychiatrist who works in a hospital in the mornings, takes scattered out-patient clinics in the afternoons, and is also re-

quired to act as consultant to a local authority and to do domiciliary visiting, cannot spend as much of his time in clinical work as he could if his work were centralized. The work of psychiatrists and other workers in the community services is of great value; but there is no more efficient way of treating a group of patients through a limited number of workers than by centralizing the patients. It costs more initially to build and equip an adequate centre; but if we take the long view, this really is 'cheaper and better for the patient'.

On the basis of these twelve propositions, we predict that there will be only a marginal reduction in the number of mental hospital beds needed. We do not attempt to quantify this prediction, because so many unknown and variable factors are involved that any statistical projection, however great its mathematical accuracy, must be based on a number of guesses; and because statistical projections provide information only on what is likely to happen, not on what ought to happen. We believe that the right answer to the present controversy is for mental hospitals to become somewhat smaller in size, but for their work to become more intensive—with all that that implies in the necessity for higher staffing ratios, higher costs, and the improvement of techniques. What is happening now is not 'the decline of the mental hospital'. It is what the World Health Organization's Expert Committee on Mental Health has described as the change from the 'classical' to the 'modern' position.[1]

In the 'classical' position, the mental hospital is the primary or the only means of psychiatric care and treatment. This is still the case in many countries today, and it was so in England until the third or fourth decades of this century. Now we are moving to the 'modern' position, where the mental hospital is one of a number of tools for the treatment of mental illness in the hands of society. The service is becoming more flexible, and, with proper selection, it should be more adequate to the needs of the patient; but the mental hospital is not outdated. It still has a vital role to play.

It is against this background of change that we describe the work of three very different hospitals—'Crown Lodge', 'Northtown', and 'Moordale'.

[1] Third Report of W.H.O. Expert Committee on Mental Health, H.M.S.O., September 1953, p. 37.

PART TWO

Three Hospitals

II

CROWN LODGE

CROWN Lodge was founded in the eighteenth century as a charitable institution for the treatment of the insane of the 'middling classes'. Funds were raised by a public subscription from the prosperous townsfolk of a fast-growing city at a time when there was no local provision save that of the workhouses, which took in 'pauper lunatics', but gave them little or no hope of treatment or cure, and the private madhouses, which charged exorbitant fees and often had an evil reputation. The proposal to found a non-profit-making hospital where middle-class patients might receive 'tender treatment' for a moderate payment was a new and enlightened one.

The new 'lunatic hospital' was administratively attached to a large general hospital, also supported by public subscription; and the link between the two continued until the National Health Service Act came into operation in 1948. The general hospital then became a teaching hospital within the Health Service; Crown Lodge was officially disclaimed by the Minister at its own request, and is now independent, being recognized as a 'registered hospital'. There are about 300 beds.

As we shall see later, it still serves the 'middling classes', and most of the patients are fee-paying. Though the cruelties of the workhouse and the private madhouse have gone for ever, and treatment in Health Service mental hospitals is free, there is still a demand for private treatment. The social context has changed, but the demand still exists.

Buildings and Distribution of Patients

As the city grew in size and confusion, the lunatic hospital began to be uncomfortably crowded in its urban setting. In the mid-nineteenth century, it was decided that it should be moved out into the country, and Crown Lodge still occupies the buildings constructed then. These are eight miles from the city and from the parent hospital, which still supplies consultant and laboratory services by contract. The hospital owns nearly three hundred acres of land, two miles from a village which is fast becoming a fashionable residential suburb; but the setting is still to date a completely rural one. There are no hospital walls, and the three buildings—the Main Block, the Male Block, and St. Barbara's, a separate hospital for elderly female patients—are set among trees and gardens, almost out of sight of each other and of the modern Nurses' Home. They might almost, from their external appearance, be Victorian private houses, being constructed of red brick with a faintly Gothic styling. The latticed windows give no indication of the fact that they are barred with iron, and not with soft lead. This is of no importance now, when ward doors are open; but it shows the care taken in the original construction. Though patients were then kept under lock and key, every effort was made to render precautions as inconspicuous as possible.

The Main Block contains the administrative offices, the hall and the canteen, and the women's wards. The latter divide to left and right—long-stay patients on one side, and short-stay patients on the other. The short-stay side is composed of accommodation for admission, treatment and convalescence. The use of the term 'ward' is avoided here, because at Crown Lodge there are no wards in either the general hospital sense of the word or in the usual mental hospital sense. The main corridor runs through the hospital, with small sitting-rooms, bedrooms and six or eight-bedded dormitories leading directly off from it; and the corridor itself is of an irregular shape, with alcoves and odd corners where patients can sit in small groups. On the long-stay side, there is a mixed unit for some 30 men and women patients, who share day accommodation; accommodation for less stable long-stay patients and geriatric accommodation. The building has two storeys, most of the bedrooms and dormitories being upstairs, and the sitting-rooms and dining-rooms downstairs. There is a semi-basement, used for offices and store-rooms.

Furnishings, curtains and carpets have been chosen with a good deal of expense, and in excellent taste. There are television sets in most of the sitting-rooms, which are small enough and numerous enough for patients to group together according to their own inclinations. Two sitting-rooms have tanks of tropical fish, and there are attractive arrangements of flowers throughout the block all the year round.

'Canteen' is again a misnomer; for the canteen at Crown Lodge is like a high-class coffee bar. It opens from 2 p.m. to 5 p.m. every afternoon to sell Espresso coffee, ice-cream, stationery, cigarettes, and confectionery ranging from bars of toffee to expensive and ornate boxes of chocolates. Many of the ambulant patients congregate here every afternoon, long-stay and short-stay patients of both sexes mixing freely, and taking their coffee either in the canteen itself or in the hall which adjoins it.

The hall is used for meetings, for regular dances (in the afternoon weekly for long-stay patients, and in the evening for short-stay patients) and for relaxation classes taken by a physiotherapist. There is an occasional cinema show, but the 16-millimetre films available have declined in popularity since the advent of television.

Most 'wards' have from 20 to 30 patients attached to them, but the ground-plan is so informal that one is seldom if ever conscious of this number at any one time. There are no locked doors in this block. These two facts taken in conjunction mean that a high ratio of nurses to patients is necessary if patients are to be kept under adequate observation. Nurses are concentrated on the admission, treatment and geriatric wards, while the convalescent ward is very lightly staffed during the day, when most of the patients are taking part in occupational therapy or other group activities.

Crown Lodge has an unusually high proportion of women among its patients, and this is reflected in the organization of the hospital. There are two female patients to every male patient, two female nurses to every male nurse (a fact which the female nurses are apt to bewail on social club dance-nights). Matron thus has twice the responsibility, in sheer numbers, of the chief male nurse. Her office is directly opposite the medical superintendent's office, and she takes her meals with the senior medical staff. The Main Block is not only the female block, but also the hospital's administrative and social centre.

The male block is only a few hundred yards away—though far enough for doctors to go by car unless they are feeling particularly energetic. It is simply the block for male patients, and serves no other purpose. The chief male nurse has his office here, and takes his meals with his deputies in the patients' dining-room. There is the same high standard of furnishing and décor, the same informality in design and arrangement; but this is not the hub of the hospital. The younger male patients sometimes complain of being 'cut off'. They are free to go to the Main Block for entertainments and the canteen, but it is always necessary for them to go to the female block—never vice versa. The chief male nurse does not have the close daily contact with the medical staff which the matron has; and male patients point to the fact that, while there is an excellent hairdressing and beauty salon for female patients, they have to rely for haircutting on the good offices of a male nurse, for whom it is a spare-time occupation.[1] These are small pointers to a difference in status between male and female patients and male and female staff.

One long-stay ward in the male block still has a locked outer door leading to an enclosed garden which is used in fine weather. The inner door leads to the rest of the wing, and is unlocked; but patients are generally not allowed to go through it unattended. Male patients and staff eat together in a large dining-room.

St. Barbara's, the hospital for about forty old ladies, is some distance away from the other two blocks, and can be reached directly from a main road. Most of the patients here are in a very deteriorated condition, often combined with extreme old age. A number of them are bed cases, some doubly incontinent. Wards are clearly defined, one ward door is kept locked, and there are closed gardens for ambulant patients. The furnishings are not of the high standard which prevails in the rest of the hospital, though they are still of good quality; and the patients, despite their physical and mental condition, are clean and well cared for.

[1] Most short-stay and some long-stay patients have parole, and can thus go out to the village barber.

The grounds also contain a modern and well-equipped nurses' home for nurses of both sexes, a new and contemporarily-designed occupational therapy centre and sheltered workshop, of which more will be said later; an out-patient clinic, held in what was designed to be a private house and is still furnished like one; a Victorian-Gothic church, now disused and kept locked (weekly church services are held in the hall for Roman Catholics and Anglicans; parole patients may go to the village churches if they wish); and a row of staff houses, now in the process of repair and modernization.

There is also a seaside annexe for 70 patients of both sexes. This is used as a centre for long-stay stabilized patients who can be allowed a reasonable degree of freedom of action and do not need an intensive level of clinical care. There is a separate matron and nursing staff; the medical superintendent visits regularly, and a general practitioner is in attendance. Long-stay patients in the main buildings are sometimes sent here for short holidays.

Patients' Fees

At first, we found it difficult to reconcile the fact that patients are required to pay a fee—the standard rate is fifteen guineas a week—with the hospital's claim to be a charitable institution, supported by public subscription; but a study of the accounts revealed that nearly half the patients paid less than the standard rate, and some paid nothing at all. Actual percentages are as shown in Table 2:

TABLE 2

Crown Lodge: Fees paid by private patients*

	%
More than standard rate	10·3
Standard rate	43·6
Less than standard rate	46·1

* As at 31st August 1958.

Patients paying more than the standard rate may receive special privileges in the type of accommodation which they occupy. Other rates are seventeen guineas, nineteen guineas and twenty-three guineas; and one patient pays a total of forty-three guineas a week for what is in effect a private suite; but no distinctions are made between those who pay the standard rate and those who pay less, or between either and the small proportion of Health Service or Ministry of Pensions cases.

There are usually thirty or forty Health Service patients, for whom the Regional Hospital Board pays £16 13*s.* 8*d.* per head per week. The exact number at any one time is liable to fluctuation, because it is computed on bed-days per year. Health Service cases are generally acute, recent, and with a good prognosis. The maximum length of stay is six months. Most patients return home after only a few weeks. We were only able to discover one patient who had to be transferred at the end of the six-month period—an alcoholic who refused to co-operate in treatment, and who went to a Health Service hospital.

There are 22 Ministry of Pensions cases—ex-Forces officers, mainly long-stay patients who have been in hospital since the end of the First World War. These patients are paid for by the Ministry of Pensions and National Insurance at the same rate as Health Service patients.

The standard rate has gone up sharply in recent years, in accord with the cost of living. In 1945, it was five guineas; by 1951, it was twelve guineas for the first six weeks, reducing to ten; in 1954, it was fourteen guineas, with no reduction; and in 1958, it rose to fifteen guineas, with the addition of an admission fee, non-returnable, of ten guineas. The patient-census in Chapter IV will show that, although these fees bias the patient-population towards the middle and upper income-groups, not all patients come from these groups. One patient was the wife of a bus driver who pointed out that five or six weeks' treatment at standard rate cost him no more than the price of a television set, and that he valued his wife's health at least as highly as the blessings of B.B.C. or I.T.V. In some circumstances, payment can be spread over a longer period than that of the actual treatment—a sort of instalment-plan appropriate to an age of high incomes and little saving. Where an elderly patient has capital and only a very small income, arrangements are sometimes made by mutual agreement for the cost of treatment to be ultimately set against the estate. Where the patient or relatives can no longer afford to pay fees at the agreed rate, the Board of Management may make substantial reductions.

Administration

The constitution of Crown Lodge is typically that of an eighteenth-century charitable trust, and the formal organization pattern devolving from it also has an eighteenth-century character, bearing little relationship to the pattern of administration in a Health Service hospital. The president of the trust is an earl —he and his predecessors have held this office for the past hundred years. There are four distinguished vice-presidents—a lord mayor, an archbishop and two bishops, holding office by virtue of invitation from the Board of Management. President and vice-presidents may attend on outstanding social occasions, but do not take an active part in policy-making or in the management of the hospital.

Trustees acquire their status by subscription—three guineas per year, or twenty-five guineas for life trusteeship. A subscription of twenty-five guineas entitles a corporate body, such as a business firm, to a trustee's vote for 20 years. There is an annual general meeting of trustees, but many do not attend, and the proceedings are largely confined to the election of the Board of Management. The last annual general meeting lasted thirty minutes. By the terms of the constitution, any twenty trustees may request an extraordinary general meeting; but this has not been done within living memory.

The Board of Management is theoretically elected from the trustees. In practice, it appears to be self-perpetuating and remarkably homogeneous. Six of the eight members are business men. Two have professional qualifications in accounting, and one is a leading solicitor in the area. There has never been a woman member, though most of the patients and staff are women. The Board of Management consists in effect of a close-knit group of shrewd and able men who have no qualifications in psychiatry or special experience of the psychiatric services, but who devote their talents voluntarily to the running of a charitable organization.

The Board meets formally once a month. Members are required by the constitution to attend at least three out of the annual twelve meetings, and if they do not do so they are not eligible for re-election.

The medical superintendent maintains weekly contact with the chairman and other members of the Board on an informal basis. It is difficult to say where his responsibilities end and theirs begin, since in so small a group there is no clear structuring of roles, and many matters are resolved after general discussion. In general, it is true to say that the medical superintendent advises the Board on matters of general policy; he makes decisions on psychiatric and clinical matters; and senior staff appointments (medical staff, matron and deputy, chief male nurse and deputy) are in effect made jointly. The Board makes the appointment, but the medical superintendent sits with them and appointments are in practice made by mutual agreement. In some instances, the medical superintendent has been asked to draw up a short list, and the Board has appointed from this.

According to the amended rules of 1950, the medical superintendent is responsible 'for the management and the entire medical and general treatment of the patients, which shall be carried out in accordance with his instructions'. He is also responsible for supplies and financial arrangements of all kinds with the exception of those involving issues of general policy, subject to the approval of the Board. In recent years, he has made arrangements for painting and decorating to be done on contract by a business firm—a saving in a small hospital, where there is not enough work to employ staff all the year round and a large number of men may be needed for short periods to complete work quickly; and he has farmed out catering to a commercial catering concern which also caters for schools, clubs and factories. This has resulted in an improvement in the food, which is excellent, the increased cost being more than offset by the catering firm's practice of bulk buying for all its agencies at a discount of from 2½ to 5 per cent.

The medical superintendent is thus an administrator; an employer for all practical purposes; and a business man. He is also a practising psychiatrist with no psychiatric superiors. He is responsible for the staff and patient relationships in the entire hospital, and for the clinical care of some 30 or 40 individual patients. We were not surprised to find that his working-time averaged 55 hours a week—and that excluded all extra-mural engagements such as domiciliary visiting, out-patient clinics, and representing the hospital at professional or academic meetings. An interesting indication of the unusual duality of his role is given by his office accommodation—a front office near the main entrance, well furnished, for interviews and the reception of relatives; and a back office, severely practical and situated in the basement, for desk-work.

Of all other senior staff, it can only be said that they bear the degree of responsibility which the medical superintendent places on them. There is no formal structuring of role, no set of powers inherent in a particular position. The matron, as the chief woman officer in the hospital, is responsible for the female nursing staff and patients. She supervises the work of the home sister, who runs the nurses' home. She is responsible for the mixed unit, the male assistant matron who deals with male patients and nurses here being on her staff. She also bears the responsibility for nurse training, both male and female student nurses coming under her supervision—and since the last point is one which affects all three hospitals, an explanation may be in place here. In mental hospitals, unlike general hospitals, the matron usually has responsibility only for female nurses and patients, and the position of the chief male nurse is theoretically of equivalent status. The General Nursing Council, however, tends to treat mental hospital matrons as though they held the sole position of authority over all staff and patients held by a matron in a general hospital, and corresponds with them on matters relating to training and status. Area nurse training officers and officials of the G.N.C. are nearly all women. A further point is that the majority of mental hospital matrons are doubly trained, being State Registered Nurses as well as Registered Mental Nurses; few chief male nurses hold the double qualifications, and the majority of those now in service hold only the qualifications of the Royal Medico-Psychological Association, which, though good of its kind, was never officially recognized by the G.N.C., and has now been superseded. The matron therefore usually has a slightly more responsible role than that of the chief male nurse; but the extent of the matron's responsibility and influence at Crown Lodge is unusually great.

We have already seen that the chief male nurse's office is in the male block, and not in the administration block. Though he joins the medical staff once a week for afternoon tea, he does not do so for lunch. (The question of who eats with whom is of particular importance at Crown Lodge, where policy-discussions are frequently carried on at meals, and there is little or no small-talk.) He has no responsibility for the mixed unit, or for the conduct of the nurses' home, though both male and female nurses are accommodated there; and he has no responsibility for nurse-training. He holds the R.M.P.A. qualifications, but is not also a State Registered Nurse. His influence is therefore confined largely to the male block, and does not extend to the hospital as a whole.

The secretary to the Board of Management is a chartered accountant, and much of his time is taken up in accounting for the administration of trust funds and the receipt of fees. He is not responsible for major issues connected with supply and purchase, which are dealt with by the medical superintendent. His office deals with pay and accounts, and he exercises some supervision over the steward's office, the steward being responsible for the day-to-day ordering of supplies[1] and for the work of his clerical staff. The head gardener and the clerk of works are responsible to the medical superintendent, and not to the secretary.

The system centralizes authority within the hospital in the hands of the medical superintendent. The way in which decision-making is divided—if it is divided at all—will depend on the individual people holding particular posts, not on the traditional structuring of the posts themselves. Such a concentration of authority makes for speedy and certain decision-making. There is only one body (the Board of Management) to be consulted; and from the Board's decision there is no appeal to a higher agency.

Since 1955, the medical superintendent at Crown Lodge has undertaken the experiment of introducing into the hospital the features of that system of mental hospital management begun in this country by Dr. Maxwell Jones at Northfield, and continued at Belmont, which is known as 'the therapeutic community'.[2] This is a rather unsatisfactory phrase, since it can be, and often is, used in other contexts. Any mental hospital is a therapeutic community in the sense that it is a human group

[1] But not food. See p. 32.

[2] See Maxwell Jones, *Social Psychiatry*, Routledge and Kegan Paul, 1955.

with a healing purpose; but the hallmarks of this particular system are quite distinct. The hospital is conceived of as a total group—doctors, patients, nurses and ancillary staff all being regarded as having a part to play in the therapeutic process. Patients and staff are organized in interlocking sub-groups which hold meetings, largely unstructured as to content. Members of a group may discuss matters of hospital policy; or their personal relationship with each other; or group relationships with other groups; or simply issues of common interest. They may make group recommendations in some cases. The purpose of this activity is to develop among both staff and patients a greater understanding of the hospital's work, and their own part in it. From an administrative point of view, this is an interesting development, particularly in a hospital with the structure of Crown Lodge. At Crown Lodge, the formal system of administration is heavily centralized. The 'therapeutic community' system attempts to reverse this tendency—to introduce a degree of democratization, so that the medical superintendent is at the centre of the community, receiving ideas and influences from a number of groups, rather than issuing orders *ex cathedra* from the top of a pyramidal structure. The two systems work in opposite directions.

The Therapeutic Community

The usual treatments for mental illness—drugs, electrical treatment (E.C.T.), insulin shock treatment, both deep and modified, and individual psychotherapy are used at Crown Lodge; but it is not possible to separate treatment entirely from administration, because to some extent the administration *is* the treatment. The system of meetings and committees is regarded as a major factor in the work of integrating sick and isolated people into a healthy community.

The main meetings in regular operation are as follows:

A. Senior Staff Meetings

1. Medical staff. (Daily, over morning coffee.)
2. Senior medical and senior female nursing staff.[1] (Daily, over lunch.)

[1] 'Senior nursing staff' is used throughout in the sense of administrative nursing staff—i.e. matron, deputy matron, assistant matron, sister tutor or their male equivalents; but not sisters or charge nurses.

3. Medical staff and senior female nursing staff. (Daily over tea.)
4. Medical staff, senior male and female nursing staff and head occupational therapist. (Weekly, over tea.)

B. Matron's Meetings

1. Matron with senior female staff and sisters. (Weekly.)
2. Matron with staff nurses. (Weekly.)
3. Matron with nurses and assistant nurses. (Weekly.)
4. Matron with male and female student nurses. (Fortnightly.)
5. Matron with domestic staff. (Fortnightly.)

C. Patients' Meetings

1. General meeting of all ambulant patients with medical superintendent, medical staff, senior male and female nursing staff, and occupational therapists. (Monthly.)
2. Entertainments Committe meeting (1 representative from each short-stay ward) with head occupational therapist. (Weekly.)
3. Catering meetings—male and female short-stay patients separately; with catering officer, medical superintendent, and other medical staff. (Monthly.)
4. Ward meetings—short-stay male and female patients separately with doctor and senior nursing staff (male or female). (Monthly.)

It will be seen that these meetings are of four different types; informal meetings for senior staff (A), formal meetings with female staff (B), formal unstructured meetings with patients (C1 and 4) and smaller structured meetings with patients which may result in direct decision-making (C2 and 3). Of them, the Entertainments Committee meeting (C2) has the most limited and direct purpose, since it meets to draw up a programme of entertainments for the following week.

Though meetings are numerous and extensive, they do not cover all staff or all patients. Ambulant long-stay patients attend only one, and disturbed patients are asked to stay on the wards, so that only patients in a fairly stabilized condition actually attend. Bed-fast patients do not participate. No patients from St. Barbara's attend. Male nurses of charge nurse level and below do not participate, and meetings for senior female staff are far more numerous than those attended by their male equivalents.

The system has been caught to some extent in transition; for this experiment is still a comparatively new one, and experience at Belmont and other hospitals which have adopted the same system indicated that it was best to move slowly, introducing meetings one at a time, rather than presenting the hospital with an elaborate system which had to be put into practice instantly. Though the initiative has come from the medical superintendent, meetings have been allowed to develop gradually, and in some cases through a demand from the group itself for some measure of formal identity. It is hoped that eventually meetings will be developed for male staff as for female staff;[1] and activity-groups are being developed on a small scale for disturbed male patients who are incapable of the high degree of verbalization required in discussion-groups.

An interesting point is the use of meal-times for staff meetings. This is 'tea and coffee sociology'—an attempt to produce an informal atmosphere for a group meeting through the provision of a meal. The meal is the ostensible purpose of meeting; the real purposes of meeting are assisted, not hampered, by the small courtesies involved. This is not, of course, a new idea. Business men commonly prefer to take their clients out to lunch rather than meeting them formally in an office setting; and schoolteachers discuss syllabuses and pupils more freely to the accompaniment of a cup of tea in the staff-room. The new element at Crown Lodge is involved in the fact that, for senior staff, every meal-time is involved. It would be quite wrong to write 'meal-break', for there is little or no relaxation, and a good deal of work is actually done during these periods. Discussion may range over such subjects as the care of individual patients; whether patients should be allowed to keep dangerous articles, such as scissors or matches; the projected opening of a new dormitory, and the selection of patients and staff for it; the new G.N.C. nursing syllabus; or clique-formation among patient groups. Strictly medical matters are usually kept to the morning coffee sessions, and at the other staff meetings discussion is pitched at a level at which nursing staff can usefully contribute.

Matron's meetings (B) were still very new during the period of the survey, and followed the appointment of a new matron

[1] This was done in the year following the survey. Details are omitted here because we wish to keep strictly to the period stated, though this means recording a transitional situation.

a month after the survey began. They produced several new ideas—a new nurses' uniform, for which nurses of each grade contributed their own ideas on style and colour; a staff social club, which opened a few weeks later; and some recommendations on details of domestic management.

The patients' general meeting (C1) is a large affair, conducted by the medical superintendent. It takes place in the main hall, and is attended by a hundred and fifty or more people in all. The medical superintendent gives out any notices of general interest, and then throws the meeting open to discussion. Patients bring up grievances, complaints or suggestions, which are then discussed with the staff. An example is given below:[1]

MRS. PARKER: I should like to ask whether something can't be done about conditions on the admission ward. I've only been here a few weeks, but I found it quite shattering—my clothes were snatched away from me, and even my personal possessions—my watch and cigarette lighter.

MRS. PRICE: I'm on the convalescent ward now, but I hated Admission. People kept me awake all night, shouting and tossing about.

MR. PENFOLD: It's worse on the male side. Some of the new patients are violent.

MR. PERRY (*complacently*): It took four nurses to hold me down when I came in. I was just *raving*.

MR. PENFOLD: I suppose it's the fault of the building; but couldn't we have cubicles with wooden partitions? Or screens?

MR. PERRY: No—there are not enough nurses to keep an eye on us all.

MRS. PARKER: I'm not complaining so much about the ward. I can see that we have to be kept under observation when we first come in. It's this awful business of losing one's personal things.

MED. SUPERINTENDENT: Mrs. Parker, how long were your clothes taken away for?

MRS. PARKER: I don't know—I was a bit muzzy at the time.

MED. SUPERINTENDENT: I think you'll find it was only for about half an hour. They weren't marked with your name before you came in, were they?

MRS. PARKER: No, they weren't.

[1] Where patients' conversations or discussions are recorded, patients have been allotted fictitious names beginning with the letter 'P', following Caudill's system. These do not in any case correspond to the real names of the people concerned, and identifying detail has been eliminated.

MED. SUPERINTENDENT: Well, in a community like this, people lose things if they're not marked. It's the same with watches and valuables—we don't return those to you, but they are kept in a safe.

MRS. PARKER: I *did* want my cigarette lighter.

MED. SUPERINTENDENT: Yes, I know, and it would probably have been quite safe with you; but suppose some other patient had got hold of it? This is an old building, and we don't want it to go up in flames. (*Laughter.*) I'm afraid there is no real alternative to putting new patients together in a small ward, even if they do disturb each other. It's only a matter of a few days, but constant observation is necessary, just in case people do something silly. The point is, if you live in a community—any community—you have to accept some restrictions. We do try to make them as few as possible.

This extract typifies the usual form of the patients' general meeting. The medical superintendent takes charge, patients raise points of complaint, and he shows the administrative necessity underlying restrictions. The medical and senior nursing staff, together with the catering officer and the head occupational therapist, are present at these meetings, and are consulted on specific issues.

The food committees are rather different. Here the patients bring up complaints about the diet, suggest alterations, and expect something to be done about it. Some complaints cannot be met. For instance, cold toast is served at breakfast—but it is impossible with the existing kitchens and kitchen staff to serve hot toast for a hundred people in the male wing all at once. (The catering officer adds that one gets cold toast in an hotel for the same reason.) The last cooked meal is at 6.30 p.m., which is too early—but it is impossible to serve it later without employing kitchen staff on shifts, which is too expensive in a small unit. The catering officer is in a rather difficult position. Placed between the catering company which employs him, the medical superintendent who is his immediate superior, and the patients, he tries to satisfy all three. A complaint is made about the sausages, and he promises to try Brown's instead of Smith's. Mr. Parkinson is tired of cheese on toast, which does not agree with him, and is promised that it will appear less frequently on the menu in future. One complaint produced a wry smile: several patients agreed that fish was served too often. On turning back to the previous week's menu, he pointed out that it had been served twice—Dover sole on one occasion and fresh salmon on the other.

Many of the points which are brought up at these meetings are similarly trivial in character; but they may not be trivial to the patients, and the medical staff listen carefully, interested perhaps less in the content of the remarks than in the underlying motivation. Even an apparently frivolous complaint may cloak a genuine one of a more fundamental nature.

Sometimes, patients are able to take a real part in decision-making in important matters. For instance, at a ward-meeting on the male wing, a point of regulations was raised:

> Mr. Pridham and Mr. Pratt were two patients who had 'outside parole' and Mr. Pridham was an alcoholic. Though there was a regulation forbidding patients on parole to go into public houses, the medical staff sometimes turned a blind eye to this practice where patients who could be trusted were involved, but those two had spent a whole evening drinking in an hotel, and Mr. Pridham had come back in a very bad condition. The medical superintendent put this situation to the group and asked for comment.
>
> The patients were almost unanimous in blaming Mr. Pratt—he was not an alcoholic himself, and he should have known Mr. Pridham's weakness. They felt that public houses and hotels should be placed completely out of bounds for all patients, to prevent this sort of situation recurring. A motion was put, seconded and carried.

In commenting generally on the operation of the committee-system, we have to question whether any real degree of decision-making can be delegated to mental patients. Clearly they can be allowed to make decisions on minor matters, such as the brand of sausages they eat; but where important issues of hospital policy are concerned, they can only make decisions if they are prepared to make the right ones. If the argument on the case of Mr. Pratt and Mr. Pridham had gone the other way—if the patients had decided that all alcoholics should be allowed to drink as much as they wished—it is very doubtful whether the medical superintendent would have accepted the group decision. Behind the apparent freedom of choice is always the ultimate veto of the man who has to carry responsibility. The medical superintendent has faith in his patients' ability to make sensible and reasonable choices. He points out that, in a hospital like Crown Lodge, many patients are people who are used to taking responsibility in normal life—business men and professional men, women who sit on voluntary committees. It can, therefore, be contended that there is in practice no conflict between the autocratic operation of the formal system, and the democratic operation of the 'therapeutic community'. On the other hand, it might be questioned whether a genuinely democratic system is possible under these circumstances. Apart from the question of an actual veto, there is the question of the patients' attitude to the doctor's wishes. Most patients like to please the doctor. They are grateful to him for treatment, sometimes pathetically so. They want his friendship and his approval, and perhaps unconsciously censor their remarks, so that he hears what they think he would like to hear. Others are paranoid; their fellow-patients hear the same complaints, relevant or irrelevant, week after week, and soon cease to take them seriously.

At the same time, it must be said that the patients like the system. It gives them a sense of dignity and purpose, removes many minor sources of irritation, and makes them feel that they are still individuals, not just cases in a psychiatrist's file.

The Medical Staff

There are six full-time medical staff: the medical superintendent, and the deputy medical superintendent; a senior hospital medical officer (S.H.M.O.); a senior registrar; and two registrars. All hold the Diploma in Psychological Medicine, with the exception of one registrar, who acts as house physician and is studying for it. There are also ten visiting consultants for other specialisms of medicine, who come from the teaching hospital to which Crown Lodge was once attached.

It is difficult to make definite statements about the allocation of duties for full-time staff. All medical staff worked throughout the period of the survey at full pressure. The senior registrar was away on a study leave for three months, and one registrar was a woman who held a part-time appointment. When she was replaced on resignation by a full-time registrar, and the senior registrar returned, the position became a little easier; but all medical staff continued to work from 8.30 a.m. to 6.0 or 6.30 p.m., with a rota for night duty in addition. During the period when the effective full-time staff was reduced the medical superintendent took a share of extra duties; but even so, this meant one night in four and one week-end in four on call for each doctor, in addition to a long day and no relaxation at mealtimes.

The Amended Rules of the hospital allow the medical superintendent and the deputy medical superintendent to undertake a certain amount of private practice, though it can be seen that they have little time available for this, and many private cases must be dealt with in free evenings and week-ends. There is a prescribed limit on the fees they may accept, 50 per cent of any fees over this sum going to the hospital accounts in each case. With this exception, the medical staff have no extra-mural work apart from a few interviews at their own out-patient clinic in the grounds—a marked contrast to the position in a Health Service hospital, where consultant staff are increasingly expected to take on sessional work at out-patient clinics, Approved Schools, and other agencies. Almost the whole of their time is devoted to intra-mural work. Since the medical superintendent deals with administration, other doctors spend virtually their whole time in clinical work on the wards and in meetings and discussions which also have a therapeutic purpose; and, as we shall show later, the patients have a significantly greater amount of clinical care (measured in time) than they do at the other two hospitals.

The Nursing Staff

The ratio of nursing staff to patients at Crown Lodge is unusually high—one nurse to three patients, as against a national average of 1 : 5·5. There are about 65–70 female nurses in the main block and St. Barbara's, and 30–35 male nurses in the male wing. It is difficult to give exact numbers, since they changed slightly at intervals due to recruitment or resignations, and there are many part-time female nurses whose time worked varies even from week to week, so that they cannot be effectively equated to full-time staff.

Female nurses work on three shifts, two by day and one by night. Part-time nurses are usually married women with families. Ensuring that all wards are provided with staff of the appropriate grade at the appropriate time is the work of the assistant matron. Nursing assistants are sometimes moved from 'ward' to 'ward' during the day to make up temporary deficiencies due to meal-times and the end of a part-time shift.

Female nursing staff worked a 48-hour week until October, when the working week was reduced to 44 hours.

Male nursing staff work on two shifts, a day shift from 8.0 a.m. to 8.0 p.m., and a night shift from 8.0 p.m. to 8.0 a.m. Although the management was willing to introduce a 44-hour working week for day staff, male nurses refused to consider this, since it involved changing to three shifts, like the female staff. A long day shift means that they have correspondingly more free days every week—usually three days, though there are some rota complications, and some overtime is worked. A few of the older male nurses have part-time jobs outside the hospital on their free days—one is a butcher, and another a taxi-driver; and they resisted any attempt to introduce a system which would make this impossible and thereby cut their total income.

Trade union activity is marked among the male nurses, and almost non-existent among the female nurses. Only one female nurse is an enthusiastic member of the Confederation of Health Service Employees, and goes regularly to Union meetings. Of the others, the full-time nurses pay their Union dues, but do not go to meetings, pointing out either that the meetings are at inconvenient times, since they are arranged to fit the shift-system on the male side, or that they prefer to spend off-duty time with their families. Part-time nurses rarely join the Union, and do not go to meetings. Of the male nursing staff, only two are not active Union members—one considered the Union 'a necessary evil' and the other said that he 'did not believe in Unions', because they were tied to one political party.

The Confederation of Health Service Employees (C.O.H.S.E.) was formed in 1946 by coalition between the Health and Welfare Workers' Union and the Asylum Workers' Union, thus integrating the trade union activity of nurses in general and mental hospitals on the eve of the National Health Service Act. At Crown Lodge, there is very little other trade union activity, and outside staff also tend to join C.O.H.S.E., though in other hospitals it is usual for them to join the National Union of Public Employees (N.U.P.E.). The total strength of the

C.O.H.S.E. branch is 130 members, all employed within Crown Lodge. The branch chairman and secretary are both male charge nurses (i.e. the male equivalent of sisters). Many of the male nurses exhibited strong feelings on the subject of trade unionism; and the way in which certain phrases recurred in conversations with them was striking. It seemed to indicate that the views expressed were more than those of the individual who was speaking—what he said was repeated from a Union meeting or a series of meetings where there had been forcible expression of these views, and some unanimity. One such phrase was in reference to the female nurses—'They all think they're Florence Nightingale, running round with a little lamp'. Female nurses, it was felt, were poor Union members. Their first loyalty was to the nursing profession, not to the Union; they rarely attended meetings, and seldom if ever contributed to discussion. They could afford to look on their work as a vocation, because they were either single women or married women with husbands to support them—they did not join in the struggle for better pay and better conditions which preoccupied the male staff, who had wives and children to support.

Another phrase much used was 'I might get sent down the drive'. Nearly all mental hospitals have long drives leading to the entrance, and being 'sent down the drive' means being summarily dismissed. The phrase was used in many mental hospitals during the insecure thirties, when there were more applicants for mental nursing posts than jobs available; but, in days of full employment and superannuation, it is now rarely used in Health Service hospitals, occurring only occasionally in conversation with a nurse of long service now nearing retirement age. At Crown Lodge, its use was marked among the older male nurses, and seems to stem from insecurity.

The 'therapeutic community' experiment involves much greater freedom for patients—unlocked doors, more parole, more movement and activity. Those nurses who remember the days of custodialism, when their chief task was to guard the patient and to prevent him from hurting himself, feel acute tensions in the demand that they should work with the patients, giving them a much greater degree of liberty of movement. Restraint means safety; freedom means risk—a nurse cannot be everywhere at once, and there is a danger that a patient may harm himself or someone else. If he does, the nurse feels that he will be held responsible—and might be 'sent down the drive'.

Married male nurses live outside the hospital estate, with the exception of the chief male nurse, his deputy, and two charge nurses. Without exception, they said that they preferred this—a hospital house would be a 'tied cottage', to be taken away from them on dismissal or retirement; and a number felt that it was important to have some life of their own outside the hospital—that they did not want their wives or families to be part of the hospital atmosphere.

Among the female nurses, nursing seems much more a way of life than a 'job' with rigidly-defined conditions and a limited contract of service. One was reminded constantly of Lord Shaftesbury's comment to the Select Committee on Lunatics of 1859—that it would always be more difficult to get male mental nurses than females, because 'the tendency of woman is to nurse'. Female nurses seem to derive a personal satisfaction from the nature of their work which was not common among male nurses; and some mentioned with particular pride the fact that Crown Lodge was a private hospital. It was not possible to determine whether this was a status-concept (a private hospital being superior to a Health Service hospital, and therefore a Crown Lodge nurse superior to a Health Service nurse) or whether it related to some innate feminine dislike of regimentation as exemplified by nationalized concerns; but while the men saw independent status as a threat to their security, and the medical superintendent primarily as an employer, the women saw independent status as an advantage, and the medical superintendent primarily as the chief doctor. Most female nurses did not seem to feel insecure because of the risks involved in the new liberal system of patient-management and were much less custodial in their attitudes.

There are several possible reasons for this. Female nurses do not generally have families to support, and the risk of dismissal weighs less heavily with them. The female wards are in the administration block, which means that the female nurses are more strongly influenced by new trends; they derive a support from the constant coming and going of medical staff, from casual conversations with them, and from the system of staff meetings with matron which is not yet paralleled on the male side.

In addition to the different attitudes of male and female nurses, there was a marked difference between younger nurses and older ones of both sexes. Like most mental hospitals, Crown Lodge recruited heavily in the nineteen-thirties, when employment was scarce, and many people who would otherwise not have done so turned to mental nursing; there was hardly any recruitment during the war period, and post-war entrants to mental nursing have been of a different type—more professional in their outlook, more conscious of the fact that they are nurses, more anxious to take single or double training with a view to promotion, more aware of their links with general nursing. There is a wide gap in attitudes and ideology between the two groups. Some older nurses still tend to look back nostalgically to pre-war days, when patients were wealthier and heavily dependent on the staff, when custodialism was enough. The younger nurses are keen to adopt new ideas and techniques, and often much preoccupied with their status as nurses. Three or four young student nurses said that they would prefer to work on the sick ward—'that's the only place in a mental hospital where you do proper nursing'. The point seemed to be that 'proper nursing' involved what might be called the technical trappings of the nursing profession—masks and white coats, oxygen cylinders and sterilizers, all the things which make up an adolescent's dream of what it means to be a nurse. Psychiatric nursing involves few trappings—though the female nurses wear a uniform, the male nurses have only a loose white coat as a source of support and group identity, and work in lounge suits. Talking to patients, inducing them to go to occupational therapy classes, accompanying them on walks, helping them to bath and shave and dress and feed themselves, does not induce the same sense of professional competence in a young nurse, and requires a more adult attitude to life.

The nurses at Crown Lodge, of both sexes and all ages, were all good nurses in the sense that they did not take advantage of the opportunities for dominance which the care of mental patients always presents. They were efficient, conscientious, gentle and polite to their patients. If we have stressed the tensions which underlie their working life, this is not because these affected the patients, who spoke frequently in praise of the nursing staff, and often added that this was a job they could not have undertaken themselves.

We regret that, in the time available for this project, it was not possible to undertake a full-scale attitude survey of nursing staff in the three hospitals. Between them, they employ over 700 nurses, and a properly-validated survey of these busy and elusive people (they are generally either fully occupied or off duty) would have been a full two-year project in itself. The major groupings, and the consensus of opinion within each group, were so clear-cut that such a survey would only have lent a superficial numerical accuracy to description, since the issues were already quite clear. We have therefore only given a generalized view, since we thought it more valuable to use the time available for an investigation of other aspects of the hospitals' working.

Ancillary Departments

Dispensing is carried out from a small dispensary in the basement. Prescriptions are made up separately for each patient, and there is no general allocation of drugs to individual wards. One dispenser works with the aid of a nursing cadet, and drugs are sent up to ward sisters or charge nurses daily. Sisters or charge nurses do not keep a supply of drugs. This individualization and lack of routine organization is possible because of the small size of the hospital, and its independent position.

Records are not centralized. Records for past patients are kept in an office, where an administrative officer deals with statistics of admissions and discharges. Again, there is very little organization—we found it necessary, when extracting material on discharged patients for the follow-up study, to work from three sets of documents at once—one kept in alphabetical order, one in order of admission, and one in order of discharge; but the hospital is so small, and the service to patients so individual, that members of staff had little difficulty in recalling from memory the salient facts about any particular patient. Case-files for present patients are kept in two other places—files for female patients in the clinical secretaries' office in the main building, and files for male patients, not in the male block but in the secretary's office attached to the out-patient clinic. Active files may be in the possession of the doctor responsible for the patient's care, and there is no record of this in the main files; so that again, we had some difficulty in the patient-census in making sure that every patient was in fact covered.

Social Work. There is no social worker at Crown Lodge. Patients commonly enter the hospital by reference from a general practitioner or a psychiatrist in private practice. On discharge, they are commended to the care of their general practitioner, and sometimes asked to return to the out-patient clinic for group or individual therapy sessions. A small fee is charged for these sessions, usually one guinea. In theory, patients may be referred to a local authority Mental Health Service for domiciliary care, but no such referral has been made within the past two years.

The medical staff point out that, since the hospital is small, they have time to handle social work problems themselves; that very few social work problems occur, since the very fact that a patient enters a fee-paying hospital usually means that he comes from a co-operative family with responsible relatives; and that, in view of the high social status of most patients, the presence of a social worker (associated in their minds with problems of poverty, and shiftless families of low social status) would be harmful rather than helpful.[1]

Occupational Therapy takes three forms—orthodox occupational therapy (i.e. rug-making, weaving, embroidery, and a number of minor interests such as calligraphy and water-colour painting); activity groups for long-stay male patients, who carry out such tasks as window-cleaning, upholstery-repairing, gardening, and house or ward-painting; and a sheltered workshop, where patients do simple repetitive forms of work and are paid for what they produce. As these three forms are quite distinct, and to some extent serve different purposes, they are here dealt with separately.

The occupational therapy block is a separate modern building in the grounds. Half is given over to the orthodox occupational therapy, and half to the sheltered workshop, the two being joined by a small lobby and a number of surrounding offices. The occupational therapy room has french windows, and in

[1] See p. 99 for further discussion of this point.

fine weather the patients work out of doors. There is a head occupational therapist and an assistant, both qualified, and they are usually helped by two students from an O.T. training school. The aim of the work is to activate patients, not primarily to produce goods. The patient may ruin the materials for his first rug or piece of weaving, and this does not matter; by the time he has learned to handle them properly, he is ready to move on to something else, to acquire another skill. The end-product is not in itself important, and occupational therapists are inclined to look askance at departments which turn out beautiful work for show. There is a great diversity in the forms of occupational therapy available for the patients at Crown Lodge, the O.T. staff taking a pride in matching the form of activity to the patient's need and interests. Some patients do very little at first, and have to be socialized gently, being introduced into small groups and persuaded to help other patients before they embark on work of their own. The patient's psychiatrist sends a 'prescription' to the O.T. staff on his first attendance, giving some indication of how he should be treated—whether he should be left alone to find his feet, encouraged into activity, set to work in a group or alone, and so on. The end-product is not important, the whole emphasis being on therapy; and the department is not expected to be self-supporting. About sixty patients of both sexes attend daily, morning and afternoons. Psychiatrists and nursing staff encourage patients to go to occupational therapy, but do not compel them to do so. There is an inducement in the fact that morning coffee is served in the occupational therapy room, but not on the wards!

In the sheltered workshop, the orientation is very different. This is under the supervision of an industrial psychologist with the help of a trained occupational therapist. Patients are encouraged to work steadily, and are paid at hourly rates. The end-product is important, since the unit competes with commercial firms in selling its products; and although it is still in the early stages, and is not yet self-supporting, it is expected that it will ultimately be so, and will probably show a profit.

At present, the main products are paper carnival hats. These have been designed by the industrial psychologist, who has broken down the work involved into a number of very simple processes, most of which are capable of being carried out by stabilized long-stay patients. The hats are up to normal production standard—each has to be perfectly formed, and strong, and sub-standard work is not accepted. They sell for £1 to £2 per gross. Stock-piling goes on during the year, and there is a big sale in the Christmas-New Year period. The industrial psychologist orders raw materials, makes contact with firms, collects the orders, and arranges delivery. At present, there is one outside worker, who handles the more complicated parts of production; but it is hoped that later, as the scheme develops, a number of outside workers can be taken in to work side by side with patients. To date, about fifteen patients, male and female, work in this unit. They are long-stay patients, stabilized, but of a fairly deteriorated type. Such patients work slowly, and few make more than ten shillings per week; but with practice at simple repetitive jobs, they should be able to earn considerably more, since with increased production the hourly rates will be increased also.

It is evident that the aim in the sheltered workshop is quite different from that in the occupational therapy room. There, competition is unknown, group activity is encouraged, and the aim is directly therapeutic. In the sheltered workshop, the patient is again being socialized—but to a work situation; and, as in a normal work situation, the natural goal is production of goods rather than improvement of social relationships, and the acquisition of new skills. For selected patients, particularly long-stay patients, this is valuable in that they are engaged on work with an outside purpose, and can regard themselves as 'having a job'—a satisfaction which normal occupational therapy precludes. The medical staff at Crown Lodge feel that there is scope for both kinds of activity, each serving a different purpose for a different kind of patient.

The male activity groups run separately under the care of a male charge nurse. These are for patients of a different type—those for whom physical activity and manual work are desirable. Some of them are disturbed schizophrenics, and some risk was inherent in allowing them to handle picks, shovels and spanners—tools which might be used as weapons by a patient of violent inclinations; but there have been no incidents of this kind since the inception of the scheme in 1956, and the staff have reported that some patients become quieter and more socialized as a result of this form of activity. An important point is that patients work together in groups—this may be an equivalent of the discussion-group for patients who are unable to verbalize easily, and who need to express themselves through gestures rather than words.

There are physiotherapy ('relaxation') classes for female patients, under the care of a qualified physiotherapist; but there is no equivalent for male patients. At the same time, there are facilities for exercise—tennis-courts, table-tennis equipment, a snooker table, a miniature golf course—which are used more by the male patients.

Amenities for Patients

Some of the amenities provided have been indicated above. There is also a small library, run by voluntary workers from the Red Cross Society; and television. For most active patients, the day revolves round the occupational therapy or sheltered workshop room, and the canteen. There is no compulsion in activity, and it was instructive to hear three of the young male patients (average age about 20) discussing this:

PETER: We could do with some organized sport. There's a table-tennis table in the main block, but we could do with one of our own. And there are no tennis-courts.

PAUL: Yes, there are.

PETER: Well, they are a long way away: and we have no racquets—though I suppose we could get them from O.T.

PATRICK: We don't really get enough exercise. My main problem here is boredom. I'm getting lazy. I've got no will-power. I don't think this is a very good preparation for life outside. I think they should organize us more.

PAUL: Well, that wouldn't be very good preparation for life outside, would it? You're supposed to stand on your own two feet.

PETER: I suppose it would be worse in the Army.

Another patient spent some time recounting the luxuries of another private hospital, where spare-time activity was highly organized. By contrast, he said, 'there's no organization here'; but he concluded his monologue about ten minutes later by saying:

'Come to think of it, at X—we were wrapped in cotton wool. The atmosphere is better here. I suppose they make you look after yourself instead of doing it all for you.'

Patient Groupings

The structure of groups for discussion and decision-making has already been described. In addition, patients group together spontaneously in their spare time. An interesting point at Crown Lodge was the extent to which these groupings were known to the medical and senior nursing staff, their advantages and disadvantages to individual patients being frequently discussed at staff meetings.

Some kinds of cliquing—particularly cliquing among alcoholics or homosexuals—are clearly antitherapeutic in character, and it is necessary in the interests of all the patients concerned that they should be broken up. Others may lead to the development of a valuable kind of group support. One such was the group of young male patients known to the older patients on the male block as 'Teddy Boys'. This was a clear-cut group of which it would have been possible at any one moment to say who was 'in' and who was 'out'. They included some leisured young men with plenty of money, at least one undergraduate, and two or three from comparatively humble backgrounds and manual occupations. They were drawn together, not by class feelings but by a common sense of youth and (so the older men said) a desire to make a noise. They talked out their problems with a remarkable frankness and some sense of responsibility. One said:

'There's a crowd of us here, all about the same age. We've all been through the same sort of experience. We can do almost as much for each other as the doctors and nurses can do for us—I think so, anyway.'

A group with a more questionable dynamic was 'The Bridge Set'—a group of middle-aged ladies, mainly the wives or daughters of professional men, which gathered every day in a particular alcove. These were long-stay patients, while the 'Teddy Boys' were short-stay patients. They seemed to be drawn together by an acute sense of social stratification and a general determination to treat Crown Lodge as a residential hotel rather than as a hospital. They refused to go to occupational therapy, because they said the acoustics were bad—'Oh, the noise'—and preferred simply to sit and talk. Much of their time was spent in gossip about the staff and the other patients, and if one member left the group for a few moments, the conversation rapidly switched to her shortcomings. The group had been asked to do some light dusting and vacuum-cleaning on the ward, and this was thought to be 'ridiculous'. As one member said, 'Of course, when we go out of here we shall go to live in private hotels, and we shall never have to do housework.'

The conversation of this group seemed so destructive in purpose that we discussed the matter with the medical staff, querying whether it would not be better to move patients in such a way as to destroy the group. They replied that they thought it was natural for women of this type to hold this kind of conversation—they would do so in the outside world; that it was better to keep the group as an entity than to spread the spirit of non-co-operation throughout the hospital; and that even this kind of group might be valuable to the patients taking part, since it did provide some kind of ego-support. It is only too easy to judge the desirability or otherwise of a group by outside standards.

These few examples may indicate the complexity of organization at Crown Lodge. There is the formal system—a highly-centralized framework with no formal structuring of subordinate roles. There is the 'therapeutic community' system, which at this time worked with varying degrees of success among different groups. There is what might be called the 'occupation-role system'—patients, doctors and nurses each with a separate role, and a common consciousness of the roles of others. The doctor, because of his professional expertise, always has a great deal of influence. There are also the informal patient groupings, which have nothing very obvious to do with the administration of the hospital, but may have a great deal to do with the progress and welfare of the individual patient.

Crown Lodge is a mental hospital providing care and treatment of an unusually high standard for a privileged group of patients. Its status as an independent hospital gives it some advantages over Health Service hospitals: there is the spur of the necessity for survival, which means ready adaptation to changing conditions; swift decision-making, because decisions are the responsibility of a small group, and do not have to be referred to a higher level; and a capacity for experimentation, typified in the 'therapeutic community' experiment, which few Health Service hospitals possess. It is possible that the 'therapeutic community' system could not be carried out in quite the same way in a Health Service hospital—certainly those Health Service hospitals which have used the method have not been able to carry it to the same lengths. In order to delegate authority, one must first possess it; and the fundamental centralization of responsibility at Crown Lodge cannot be paralleled within the Health Service.

At the same time, there are inherent disadvantages in independent status. Crown Lodge is to some extent isolated from the Health Service, and cut off from the developing community services. Northtown and Moordale provide a strong contrast in this respect, and the implications of this isolation will be further discussed in Chapter V.

III

NORTHTOWN

THE main buildings at Northtown were constructed in the same decade as those at Crown Lodge, but in a very different tradition; for while Crown Lodge has always served a somewhat privileged section of society, Northtown was founded as a county asylum for the under-privileged—the 'criminal and pauper lunatics' of the mid-nineteenth century.

The hospital was once situated in the country, but the spreading industrial areas soon engulfed it, and buildings of red brick and grey stone have become virtually indistinguishable under successive layers of grime. There are two main blocks, each with its own grounds and bounded by a high stone wall. Though the massive iron gates are always open, their presence is an additional reminder that Northtown was built primarily with a custodial purpose, and the initial impression is a grim one.

Before 1930, this was 'The —shire County Asylum, Northtown'. It was administered by a County Asylums Board inclined to parsimony and slow to accept change. The overall administration was far from progressive; and Northtown had one medical superintendent who claimed with pride that he ran the cheapest asylum not only in the Board's area but in the whole country.

The Mental Treatment Act of 1930 introduced some changes. The County Asylums Board became the County Mental Hospitals Board. The asylum became 'Northtown County Mental Hospital'. At first, the change was largely a terminological one, for although the Act made it possible for patients to enter mental hospitals voluntarily, not one bed was made available for voluntary patients in any of the Board's hospitals between 1930 and 1932. The central Board of Control made representations, pointing out that every other authority in England had turned over beds for this purpose, and some, by 1932, were admitting as many as 45 per cent of their patients on a voluntary basis. The County Asylums Board then agreed to admit 5 per cent of their patients on this basis, and plans for special units for voluntary patients were put in hand.

At Northtown, two small modern villas were constructed, and a separate neurosis unit was planned, though this was not completed before the outbreak of war in 1939. These special provisions concerned only a small proportion of patients, and they were necessary precisely because the standards in the rest of the hospital were so low. Patients suffering from a mild degree of neurosis could not be expected to come willingly to the ordinary wards, nor to benefit from being there.

In 1948, the National Health Service Act brought more changes. The County Mental Hospitals Board ceased to exist, and Northtown, like any other hospital in the area, came under the aegis of the Regional Hospital Board. Because of its size—there are 2,750 beds—it was not combined with other hospitals in a hospital group, but had a Hospital Management Committee of its own. Its name changed again—now it was not a county asylum, or a county mental hospital, but simply 'Northtown Hospital', part of the psychiatric provision for England and Wales.

The change of title gave Northtown at least a theoretical parity of esteem with other hospitals—something which it had never had before; and during the past eleven years much has been done to translate this into reality. More money has been made available. There is a great deal of new equipment, including an electro-encephalogram, X-ray apparatus, and a good up-to-date operating theatre. Specialist officers have been appointed, and staffing ratios improved. Wards are being systematically upgraded—though the premises are so vast and the dirt re-forms so quickly that this is a thankless task, and the results are only immediately apparent on the smaller wards.

A hospital as large as Northtown cannot be changed overnight, or even in a few years. The duality of provision constantly strikes the observer. At one moment, one is in the setting of a good modern hospital, with pastel-painted walls and chintz curtains as pleasant adjuncts to modern and efficient equipment. At the next, one is plunged back into the 'asylum' atmosphere of locked doors, long stone corridors, and large bare wards containing a hundred or more patients, many of them actively dementing. The best and the worst of the mental hospital world exist here side by side. It will be a long time before the change is complete and 'Northtown Hospital' has overcome 'the asylum'.

This is not the fault of the present-day staff, or of the Management Committee, or of the Regional Hospital Board. It is the result of built-in disadvantages: a long tradition of cheap custodial care; a catchment area which includes some of the poorest and roughest quarters of the industrial North; buildings designed by the Victorians for the reception of 'the lower classes'; high maintenance costs, due to out-of-date buildings and city grime; difficulties in nursing recruitment, due to the attractions of near-by industry; and above all, the problems of large size and scattered units.

The Main Building

Outside, the main building looks bleak and unimpressive. This is largely because visitors see it from what was once the back entrance. The original main entrance led directly into the superintendent's quarters—an interesting relic of the days when the patients were admitted direct to the medical superintendent's presence, and the staff used the back door. Now the medical superintendent lives in a house in the grounds, his quarters have become a ward, patients are generally admitted directly to the relevant wards by side doors, and the former 'servants' entrance' is the entrance to the administrative block. A whole history of mental hospitals might be written around facts such as these, and their implications in changing administrative patterns.

Male and female wards branch off to right and left from the administrative offices. They vary in size from 26 patients on what is still called the 'male refractory ward' to 80 on a ward for long-stay stabilized women patients. The admission wards are fairly small, having 35–40 beds; and they have a high staff ratio because of the necessity for keeping new patients under observation—usually six nurses at any one time in each ward. The large number of wards means that a considerable degree of classification of patients is possible, and patients are assigned to particular wards on a basis of the need for observation and nursing care rather than on diagnostic criteria. A patient who needs constant observation might thus be put on the sick ward or kept in the admission ward because these wards have a ratio of one nurse to six or seven patients, while a ward for long-stay stabilized patients might have only two nurses for 70 or 80.

Many wards are typical mental hospital wards of the older type—large rectangular day-rooms with high ceilings and a coal fire at either end protected by a heavy guard; dining-rooms either separate, or at one end of the day-room; long dormitories with beds on both sides, and sometimes down the middle as well; a series of smaller rooms, once used as padded cells, but now mainly converted to offices, store-rooms or single bedrooms. A few padded rooms are still kept foı patients who, in a manic fit, might do harm to themselves or to other people, but these are used only for short periods. Each instance of use, and its duration, must be recorded by the nurse in charge; and seclusion is increasingly being replaced by sedation. On many wards, the allotment of a single room is a much sought-after privilege—the patient regards it as a small home of his own, where he can spread his few possessions.

Each ward consists of this series of rooms, and is cut off from the rest of the hospital by a heavy wooden door with a double lock, and a stretch of stone corridor or staircase. Eleven wards in the main building are open and thirteen are kept closed, patients only being allowed in and out under nursing escort and in groups for specific purposes.

On many wards, there are no lockers for patients, and they have nowhere to keep their personal possessions. Photographs or sweets or toilet articles which are left lying about tend sometimes to disappear; and the women patients, particularly those who 'work out', often equip themselves with holdalls or shopping bags into which they cram everything they own—not only the small possessions mentioned above, but also shoes, hats, underclothing and other articles of considerable bulk.

These holdalls are carried wherever they go—to work, to meals, to the cinema or the library. The men cram their pockets, and a few have small suitcases or ditty-bags.

All wards have television sets and radios in the day-rooms; and on the female side, special 'television nurses' are employed —married women who work part-time, and who stay in attendance on the patients during television hours, thus relieving the regular staff.

The rehabilitation ward for women patients, and the two villas for parole patients, have quite a different atmosphere, largely because they are small and the basic architecture does not express a custodial idea. The rehabilitation ward is situated in what was originally the medical superintendent's house —part of the main hospital block, but still with some of the characteristic informality of a private house. The bedrooms—containing four or six beds—are upstairs, and downstairs, the drawing-room and dining-room of the old house have been converted into patients' lounges. The patients can make tea for themselves, though unfortunately the old kitchens have been removed and they cannot do their own cooking; but there is plenty of drying-space for their personal washing in the basement, and they can get used to the sensation of living in a private house, adjusting themselves to a small domestic community, before leaving the hospital for normal home life.

The male and female villas for parole patients are small modern bungalow-type buildings, each for about 50 patients. These are open wards.

There is also a modern villa for tubercular patients of both sexes. At the time when this was visited, there were 22 male patients and 10 females, but the numbers and the proportions vary. This is also run on permissive lines. Patients have a joint day-room, and sometimes share dining accommodation. A chest physician visits weekly, and holds an 'out-patient clinic' for patients from other wards who are convalescent from tuberculosis or suffering from a mild infection.

The Annexe

This block, which is devoted exclusively to the care of long-stay patients, is the biggest in the hospital. It houses 1,700 patients, male and female, in wards which stem off from a rigidly straight main corridor. A visitor may stand at one end, and look down successive receding arches to the door at the far end, exactly a quarter of a mile away. Every bed is occupied, and there are very few discharges except by death, so that the population is very nearly static.

As in the main building, there is a rigid distinction between the sexes: one-eighth of a mile of male wards, one-eighth of a mile of female wards.

Most of the wards are very large—80 to 120 patients per ward is common. One female ward has 141, including 57 epileptics. The female geriatric ward has 130, of whom 18 are completely bed-fast, and 20 regularly incontinent.

The smallest ward in the Annexe is the male refractory ward, where there are only 34–36 patients; but these are patients who need to be kept under constant observation, since they are all capable of suicide or violence. There are six nurses on duty, but constant vigilance is necessary. The charge nurse on this ward said that a good nurse developed an instinct for the detection of danger. He was unable to associate this with any particular variation in the patient's behaviour, but he knew when to observe a particular patient minutely, and when it was safe to relax his guard a little. A nurse who did not develop this sense, however great his technical skill, was of no use on such a ward.

Thirteen wards on the Annexe are open. From these, patients go out in working parties to farms or gardens (men) or to cleaning and laundry work (women). All wards have television sets and there is some occupational therapy, but there is little social activity—these are nearly all deteriorated patients, many of them dementing, and incapable of more than a very limited response. There are nursing offices for both the female and the male side, run by an assistant matron and an assistant chief male nurse respectively. Some medical staff are wholly engaged in the Annexe, but others work there on a sessional basis, spending the rest of their time in other parts of the hospital. There is one full-time consultant in the Annexe, who deals with administrative as well as clinical work.

Nursing staff do not remain in the Annexe, but work on a rota in different parts of the hospital in turn. Both the matron and the chief male nurse consider that permanent work in this block would be too depressing for staff, and that they need the stimulus of change.

The Neurosis Unit

This unit, as already indicated, is intended purely for short-stay patients suffering from the milder types of mental disorder, and was constructed in order to keep such patients from the necessity of participating in the asylum-type life of the main building and the Annexe. It was completed in 1940, but used as a military hospital during the war. Subsequently, it was redecorated and refitted, and opened for its original purpose in 1950. Here there are no closed wards, and patients have freedom of movement.

A small lounge is kept for the reception of new patients. This, like the rest of the unit, is well decorated and furnished. The social worker attached to the unit commented, 'Patients are usually terrified when they first come in, and this room reassures them.'

As with the villas and the female rehabilitation ward, there is a pleasant, informal atmosphere which contrasts sharply with the 'asylum' atmosphere of the rest of the hospital. This is difficult to convey in words, and seems to arise from a number of factors: modern design and decoration; small rooms; modern fireplaces and doors—the latter unlocked; casual movement in and out, the sight of patients carrying out small domestic activities in spontaneously-formed groups, making tea, arranging flowers, standing round the piano while one of their number plays; the fact that the patients are not suffering from the grosser forms of psychiatric disorder—they wear their own clothes, look 'normal', and there is a good deal of chatter and laughter.

Our initial impression was that the patients in the neurosis unit were of a higher social status than those in the main building and the Annexe, and we wondered whether the noticeable difference in atmosphere was partly due to social privilege; but an analysis of the patient-population[1] showed no significant difference in social status between patients in this unit and those

[1] See Chapter V.

in the others. The patients do not come from more well-to-do homes, have more influential relatives, or have more acquired social graces. The impression is, we think, due to their youth, the mild degree of mental disorder, and the feeling of hopefulness in a unit where every patient is free to discharge himself if he wishes. No one has been in hospital very long, and everyone expects to go home soon.

Although the neurosis unit has between 40 and 50 patients, it could easily house twice that number, and there appears to be a difficulty in finding suitable patients for a unit of this nature. One of the medical staff suggested that general practitioners in the area were not sufficiently aware of the kind of facilities offered, preferring to keep patients at home, or to send them to out-patient clinics, even when home conditions were unsuitable. He felt that the old reputation of Northtown as a county asylum kept patients away, and that it was not generally realized that the neurosis unit operated quite separately at the patient-level. Such a unit, he thought, stood a better chance of public acceptance if it were spatially separated from the parent hospital, though this of course would increase difficulties of administration in some ways.

The Northtown neurosis unit is not administered as an independent unit on the staff level. Three psychiatrists attend, each for the treatment of his own patients, but none of them has a responsibility for the unit as a whole, this responsibility remaining with the medical superintendent. There is no doctor in full-time attendance. Nursing staff, following the policy described earlier, are not permanently attached to one unit, but move about from one part of the hospital to another. This policy operates to the benefit of the long-stay wards, but means that nursing staff sometimes carry over custodial attitudes more appropriate to the Annexe than to this very different sphere.

It seems possible that a policy of treating the neurosis unit as an autonomous unit at staff as well as patient-level might increase its efficiency. One psychiatrist who felt a definite responsibility for the unit's success might well work up contacts with local general practitioners, and keep the unit working at full strength for the type of patients it was designed to treat—there is certainly no lack of such patients, and the unit is potentially an excellent one. A group of nurses permanently assigned to the unit could be made aware by daily contact with a psychiatrist of the special attitudes and techniques appropriate to nursing patients of this type. Such a policy, however, would operate in favour of the neurosis unit against the interests of the rest of the hospital. The question of how far priority should be given to short-stay patients at the expense of long-stay patients is a difficult one, and there is no easy solution. The patients in the neurosis unit already have many advantages in comparison with the patients in the Annexe and the main building, and this allocation of special staff might well be unjustifiable.

Most of this report on Northtown has been filled so far with descriptions of the small special units for short-stay patients. This is because they have special features which deserve comment; but it should be remembered that the total number of patients in the two villas, the female rehabilitation ward, the tuberculosis villa and the neurosis unit does not exceed 250—and there are 2,750 patients in the hospital. Of these, nearly 1,000 are on closed wards, many of them of the old asylum type. In all, there are probably not more than 450 or 500 short-stay patients at any one time, as against more than 2,000 long-stay. The discharge rate for 1958 was 97 per cent, which is high; but this means that a small proportion of short-stay beds turned over several times, while the great bulk of the hospital population was unchanged.

If one thinks in terms of admissions, these small modern units play a large part in the hospital's activity, because many patients pass through their hands. If one thinks in terms of the standing population at any one time, the picture is a very different one. Northtown has a huge chronic population, many of whom will probably remain there for the rest of their lives.

Administration

As already indicated, Northtown has its own Hospital Management Committee, and is not part of a hospital group because of its size. This operates under the Regional Hospital Board, which appoints the Chairman. Of the nineteen members of the Management Committee, four are medical practitioners; six are justices of the peace; six represent Trade Union and Co-operative interests; and two are businessmen. Apart from the representatives of the Medical Council, the Executive Council and the Regional Hospital Board, almost all are active in local government—there are two aldermen and five councillors. There are four women, of whom two are justices of the peace, one is an alderman, and one is a councillor.

The members of the Management Committee are thus people with a long tradition of local public service. With the exception of the medical members, there are no representatives of the professions.

There are four standing sub-committees for special purposes: Establishments, Finance, General Purposes and Catering. An ad hoc committee deals with Building and Planning; and there is a Joint Contracting Committee with another mental hospital of similar size in the neighbourhood. This last committee is able to carry out bulk buying for a total of about five thousand patients with considerable financial saving.

The Management Committee takes an active part in the formulation of policy, and in the appointment of officers. Senior medical officers are appointed by the Regional Hospital Board, but a wide range of appointments is in the hands of the Management Committee, which also deals, as indicated, with a number of other important issues at policy level. The medical superintendent advises the Committee, and they have much confidence in his judgements; as at Crown Lodge, it is difficult to state where his sphere of authority ends and the Committee's begins, since this is a matter dependent on personality and mutual agreement.

The medical superintendent at Northtown said in conversation, 'I'm running five hospitals—the male and female sides of the main building and the Annexe, and the neurosis unit.' This statement expresses two fundamental facts about Northtown succinctly.

First, the medical superintendent runs the hospital. His range of authority is greater than that of medical superintendents in many mental hospitals, and the pattern of administration is a highly centralized one. The medical superintendent has the confidence of his Committee; and in day-to-day management, secretary, matron, chief male nurse and consultants all defer to his experience and authority. He is a constitutional monarch—but still a monarch rather than a team leader.

Second, the male and female sides of the hospital operate separately. There is not the unevenness of status noticed at Crown Lodge, for there is no great difference in proportion between men and women patients, and administrative headquarters is in the main building, which has a male and a female wing. Administrative offices for the chief male nurse and matron are sited on these wings, and are roughly equidistant from the medical superintendent's office on the main corridor. To use another analogy: like two brigades in one army, they have their independent lines of authority, and there is no clear means of liaison, save through the High Command.

The one point of contact—the nurses' training school—is also a point of potential friction. The General Nursing Council deals with the matron on matters relating to training and the tutors' salaries, and regards the matron as the tutors' superior within the hospital—a position which she does not hold in fact; for both tutors are men, and in practice responsible to the chief male nurse.

Matron is responsible for female nursing staff, ward-maids, and for the running of the nurses' home. There is no home sister, and she spends much time on staff welfare problems. Dining-room staff and officers' maids, including matron's own maid, come under the supervision of the catering officer.

The chief male nurse deals only with male nursing staff. There is no accommodation for male nurses in the nurses' home—ten single male nurses sleep in the neurosis unit, and others in single rooms on individual wards. There are 70 staff houses for married male staff.

The work of the secretary's department is fairly clear-cut. He is secretary to the Management Committee. A large staff deal with matters of pay, accounts, supplies and records—all complex matters in a community of 2,750 patients and about 700 staff, with an annual expenditure of well over three-quarters of a million pounds. This is a busy and well-organized department at an executive level. It does not, in general, deal with matters of policy, which are the prerogative of the Management Committee and the medical superintendent. The relationships between medical and lay administration appear to be good—

they operate on well-defined channels; and the individuals concerned have achieved a *modus vivendi* which does not appear to cause undue friction.

Medical Staff

The total medical staff, including the medical superintendent and the deputy medical superintendent, numbers 22. There is one vacancy for a junior house medical officer. Staff appointments are as follows:

Consultants	6
S.H.M.O.s	3
Sen. Registrars	3
Registrars	3
J.H.M.O.s	7
	22

In addition, there is a visiting neuro-surgeon and a visiting chest physician.

The overall ratio of resident medical staff to patients is 1 : 130, but this ratio does not express the real situation, for several reasons:

(*a*) The medical superintendent, the deputy medical superintendent and the consultant in charge of the Annexe have a heavy burden of administrative work.

(*b*) All consultant staff have a great deal of extra-mural work —domiciliary visiting, out-patient clinics, sessional work at Approved Schools, and court appearances in connection with criminal proceedings. The extension of the psychiatrist's work into the community has many benefits to the community, and has done much to break down the mental hospital's sense of isolation; but it means that in practice the bulk of in-patient clinical care is done by junior medical staff.

(*c*) Since the medical staff is so large, and the annual period of leave due to each doctor is six weeks, the equivalent of two doctors' work per year is spent in holidays.

It is estimated, therefore, that a more realistic ratio would be 1 doctor : 200 patients; but the allocation of medical time is not of course evenly divided between all patients. Our survey of the average medical clinical time spent with each patient (see p. 135) gave a figure of 29·9 minutes per week per short-stay patient, and 5·7 minutes per week per long-stay patient.

The treatment orientation at Northtown is almost wholly organic; and indeed it is difficult to see how psychodynamic or psychoanalytic methods could be employed in the time available, for even the short-stay patient can only expect to see his psychiatrist for half an hour a week, while the medical care of long-stay patients must be minimal. At the same time, Northtown is able to compensate for this lack of facilities for individual clinical care by means of excellent facilities for diagnosis and laboratory investigation.

All the consultants possess the D.P.M., but of the sixteen junior doctors (and they, as we have seen, are responsible for the bulk of in-patient work) only two have a D.P.M., and one is studying for it. One doctor has studied psychoanalysis in Vienna. The rest are qualified medical practitioners, but not (except by experience) qualified psychiatrists. The D.P.M. is not at present a registrable medical qualification, and some mental hospitals still recruit doctors who do not possess it and may have no intention of undergoing a special course of psychiatric study. In a hospital where the ratio of doctors to patients is low, it may be difficult for a doctor to secure the necessary time for study.

Medical meetings occur twice a week. One of these is confined to the six consultants, and discusses matters of day-to-day policy under the chairmanship of the medical superintendent. The other is for all members of the medical staff. Because of its size, it is difficult for this to become an open discussion-group, with all members taking part, and its time is generally taken up with (*a*) notices given out by the medical superintendent; (*b*) discussion of general clinical issues, in which senior staff, who tend to sit together, take the major part; and (*c*) the interviewing of three or four individual patients to be considered for leucotomy operations.

Two doctors have experimented with group psychotherapy on a small scale, and one uses the psychoanalytic method in certain cases; but the conditions of work for the medical staff at Northtown are such that an organic form of treatment is the only one they are in a position to offer in most cases. It is quicker to give a patient E.C.T. than to make an attempt at understanding his personal problems—one takes only a few minutes, while the other would take several hours of personal interviewing a week. One is a technique which can be learned fairly quickly by a qualified medical practitioner; the other demands a great deal of knowledge and experience, and constant professional discussion with colleagues. It is not suggested that psychodynamic methods are necessarily superior to organic methods—the psychiatric profession is itself divided on this matter; but at Northtown, as at most large mental hospitals with small staffs, the medical staff have no choice.

Nursing Staff

The total nursing staff is 522 (part-time nurses equated to full-time), which gives an overall ratio of one nurse to 5·25 patients. There is a shortage of 67 nurses on the male side. On the female side, there is no outstanding shortage, but many part-time nurses are employed—in the Annexe, nearly all nurses under the rank of sister are part-timers.

The chief male nurse thought that the staff shortage on the male side was due to low wage-levels. In an industrial area, where people of the calibre of the average male nurse can earn very much higher wages than a male nurse does, he thought that some men might be attracted to the work for its own sake, but that their wives would not accept smaller pay packets and would influence them against it. Staff houses were a great advantage. Male staff did not look on a hospital as a 'tied cottage' (the attitude found at Crown Lodge) but as a cheap house within easy reach of work which would be maintained for them. The chief male nurse thought that if there were more hospital houses or flats available, he could solve his staff shortage.

The position on the female side was easier. Matron had recruited some nurses—ten or fifteen—from abroad; and the wives of male nurses living on the hospital estate often came in for part-time service. Both male and female nurses work the 'long day'—a single day shift of 12 hours and a night shift of 12 hours.

The matron and the chief male nurse are both responsible for nursing in the main building and the Annexe. A considerable amount of time is taken up in getting from one to the other; and both felt that their own work would be easier and the staff shortage lessened if their patients were centralized—i.e. if, for example, all female patients were moved to the present Annexe, and all male patients to the present main building; but it was interesting that neither had thought out the advantages and disadvantages of this suggestion in detail. They felt that if this was advisable as a matter of general hospital policy, it would be suggested by the medical superintendent and put up to the Management Committee. Since this had not been done, they assumed that there were overriding considerations which made it impossible—but did not feel that this was a sphere of decision-making in which they could take part, or even bring forward points for discussion.

The general structure of the nursing staff is roughly the same as at Crown Lodge, though there are less doubly-trained nurses —only four on the female side—and less single women are employed. Male nurses here also referred to the female nurses as 'Florence Nightingales', and complained that they took little part in trade union activity.

Among the male nurses, there seemed less sense of insecurity than at Crown Lodge. The fact that they are prepared to accept hospital houses, and that these are sought after, is an index of their feeling of security in the Hospital Service.

Nevertheless, trade union activity is strong among the male staff at Northtown. The Confederation of Health Service Employees is the strongest Union, having over 500 paid-up members. Administrative staff join the National and Local Government Officers' Association, and outside and maintenance staff join the National Union of Public Employees. The branch secretary of C.O.H.S.E. represents all three Unions on the Joint Consultative Council.

When the Ministry of Health circular relating to the 44-hour week for mental nurses was published, the matron and the chief male nurse stated that hours of work could not be reduced without a 10 per cent increase in staff. Since this could not be obtained, no immediate plans for the introduction of the 44-hour week were made. The Branch Committee of C.O.H.S.E. then complained that they had not been consulted by the Management Committee and the medical superintendent, and stated that this was a matter for the Joint Consultative Council. After some heated discussions among themselves, they threatened a work-to-rule unless the 44-hour week was introduced immediately.

A meeting of the chairman and secretary of C.O.H.S.E. with the Management Committee and the medical superintendent was arranged. This does not seem to have been a regular meeting of the Joint Consultative Council (which would have necessarily included representatives of the other occupational groups in the hospitals, such as technical staff, administrative staff, and outside staff) and was dealt with separately as a matter only concerning C.O.H.S.E.

At this meeting, the Management Committee agreed in principle to the introduction of the 44-hour week, pointing out that this would involve a switch to the 8-hour day. The Management Committee also pointed out that this could only be implemented if the existing staff shortage of 67 on the male side were overcome, and agreed to advertise for additional male nurses.

There were 60 replies to these advertisements, nearly all of them from men over 50 years of age. A number were interviewed, and only four were found to be acceptable. The situation thus remained unchanged.

Meanwhile, the male nurses had discussed among themselves the implications of the shorter day. Some liked the 'long day' system because it gave them more whole days of duty, and they had outside work which supplemented their income. Others wanted the unbroken free time because their wives were part-time nurses, and they looked after the children while their wives worked. Eventually they passed a resolution rescinding their previous decision to press for the 44-hour week—and the *status quo* has been maintained. This was in direct opposition to the views of the C.O.H.S.E. secretary and chairman, both of whom pressed for the introduction of shorter hours on the grounds that no nurse could work a 12-hour day without strain, and without loss of sensitivity to the patient's needs.

On the whole, nursing staff seemed contented at Northtown, and many described it as 'a happy hospital' in spite of the recent dispute. Perhaps the groups involved are large enough for personal animosities to play a small part. Nursing staff seem to like the feeling that they are part of a nationalized undertaking and thus practically 'civil servants'. This gives them a sense of security. Another source of contentment, paradoxically enough, springs from the fact that much of the care at Northtown is still of a custodial nature. We noticed that the only marked signs of tension among nursing staff occurred in the neurosis unit, where patients have a degree of liberty to which custodially-trained staff are not accustomed.

Ancillary Departments

Because of its large size, Northtown can employ a number of specialist officers and set up specialist departments, where a small hospital has to rely on outside services. Northtown is the only hospital of the three which has its own well-equipped operating theatre, its own laboratories, and its own electro-encephalogram. Physical tests are carried out as routine here, while at the other two hospitals they involve a special journey to a general hospital, an ambulance, and a nurse as escort. The services for the physical care of patients and for psychiatric treatment by organic means thus reach a high level of efficiency.

Psychologists. There are two full-time psychologists, who have their own offices in the neurosis unit. They carry out diagnostic tests and do a good deal of research work, some of which has been published in the psychiatric journals.

Social Workers. Three full-time social workers deal with the social problems of in-patients. Northtown is situated in an area where the local authorities are fairly jealous of their rights under section 28 of the National Health Service Act, and the social workers are expected to concentrate on in-patient care, handing over cases to local authority mental welfare officers on discharge. This is usually done, and there is a good liaison with the local authority workers. Two social workers share an office in the main building. They are also responsible for the Annexe, but are very conscious that much more work could be done there if time permitted. One said, 'I dread going over to the Annexe—I know that when I get there, I shall be there for the rest of the day. All the patients and half the nursing staff will have problems lined up for me.' The problems of the short-stay patients are so time-consuming that there is little time for the less pressing problems of long-stay patients.

The third social worker is fully occupied in the neurosis unit. Although there are only 40–50 patients there at any one time, there is a rapid turnover, and many of these patients have difficult problems which have contributed to their mental breakdown. These are mostly patients under 40. Many of them have employment problems, problems connected with the care of young children, hire-purchase problems. The social worker commented that if a new television set was not paid for in hard cash, it was often paid for in mental stress—the inability to keep up hire-purchase payments was a contributory factor in breakdown.

The three social workers all have previous experience of social work over a number of years, and one has attended a short university course. None of them has a formal social work qualification, though the hospital designates them 'psychiatric social workers'. Most of their work consists of taking social histories (this may include domiciliary visiting to elicit information from relatives), and dealing with pensions, insurance and employment problems. There is little time or opportunity for social case-work. All three felt that they would like to have more time for individual patients, and that there was a great deal of work in which they merely skimmed over the surface for lack of time.

Records. There is a well-designed Records Department, with an administrative staff of four. All case-records are kept up to date, filed and cross-indexed, and any one can be located at a moment's notice. We spent some time working in this department on patients' case-files, and found that it worked at a maximum efficiency.

Library. There is a full-time librarian—a graduate—who runs what is in effect a branch of the County library. The library is a separate building, entered from the drive, which contains a reading-room and an excellently-stocked lending section. Two patients act as assistants in issuing books, classification, and general maintenance. The library is available for both staff and patients, and includes a wide range of reading matter, while special requests can be met through the national library system. The librarian also runs art classes for patients, and is interested in using the library as a means of education, not merely of entertainment.

Occupational Therapy. It is difficult to give a general picture of what O.T. activities take place, because this work is scattered through the hospital. There is an O.T. unit in the main building, one in the Annexe in which the work merges about imperceptibly into utility work for the hospital, and one in a sitting-room in the neurosis unit. Although a great deal of work goes on at any one time, the hospital is so large and the patients are so numerous that many patients are only able to attend for one day or even half a day per week. The work done is of a fairly orthodox type—lampshade-making, basket-work, rug-making, knitting, sewing, embroidery. The patients who attend appear to enjoy it—while at Crown Lodge, attendance at O.T. was encouraged by the doctors and resisted by some of the patients, facilities are so limited that it is rather a privilege to attend at Northtown. This may make the work more pleasant for the O.T. staff.

In the neurosis unit, O.T. work is linked closely with medical care. The psychiatrist sends a prescription card to the occupational therapist; and the occupational therapist keeps a record of the patient's progress which the psychiatrist can consult.

Chaplaincy Services. Northtown has two full-time chaplains—one Church of England and one Roman Catholic—in addition to visiting Free Church ministers and a visiting rabbi. Each of the full-time chaplains has his own large Church, and they work in liaison with the parish clergy when patients are admitted and discharged.

Physical Training. There are two male and two female P.T. officers, all working full-time. They organize indoor physical training, remedial exercises, Health and Beauty classes, and outdoor sports including football, cricket and hockey. The hospital runs its own football and cricket teams for men, in which the P.T. officers and occasionally other members of the staff play beside the patients.

Patient Activities

In addition to the activities noted above, many patients are engaged during the day on utility activities—cleaning the wards, the windows and the corridors. It is still a common sight to see a deteriorated patient marching up and down with a 'jumbo'—a heavy polishing pad with which, little by little, he succeeds in giving a high polish to a linoleum-covered floor. Patients who can leave the wards are engaged in groups on other forms of employment. Some male patients work on the farm, or in the gardens; others go to the carpenter's shop or the cobbler's shop. Female patients may go to the laundry or the sewing-room, and some go under the care of nurses to clean and tidy male wards.

This work reduces the cost of running the hospital, since, although patients generally work much more slowly than outside workers, and need supervision, they do between them a good deal of unskilled work. Since most patients were manual workers before entry to hospital, such a work-situation is 'normal' for them, and a hospital life which left them unlimited leisure would not be therapeutic in character; but though such work may be well suited to some patients' needs, it does not suit all. There is always a danger that it will be undertaken for the sake of the hospital, not for the sake of the patient. The staff at Northtown have therefore tried to find in the neighbourhood work which could be carried out by patients under 'sheltered workshop' conditions. This is not an easy matter, since several considerations must be taken into account: Northtown is in an industrial area, and local trade union interests must be conciliated; patients must not be given work which could be done under normal employment conditions by outside workers. Again, the hospital economy depends partly on patient-labour. Any work which is taken on must not carry such a high rate of pay that it will attract an overwhelming proportion of patients from utility work, for which they are paid the relatively low hospital rate. The kind of work must therefore be carefully selected. It must be of a simple, routine nature; it must be wage-producing; but the wage must not be so high that it would be possible for an outside worker to live on it, or even so high that it will induce many mental patients to be dissatisfied with the rewards of utility work.

One such form of work has been discovered to date—stripping down wire cables for the Post Office. This is a slow and tedious job for which it is not possible to find outside workers, since the rates of pay involved cost more than the scrap value. However, the scrap value is considerable, and mental patients, working at low rates of pay, make it an economic proposition. Only a few long-stay patients have so far participated in this activity.

Spare-time activities are varied. In addition to the forms of sport mentioned, and the ubiquitous television sets, many of the male wards have billiard tables, darts, dominoes, and other games. There is a regular dance and whist drive on Tuesday nights in the main building which involves about 200 patients. Cinema shows for all ambulant patients are given weekly in both the main building and the Annexe. The library provides books—parole patients go and choose their own, or stay to read papers or journals in the reading-room; patients on closed wards have books brought to them, a trolley-full at a time. There is a large canteen near the entrance to the main building, and a small one in the Annexe—though these are shops rather than cafés, as conditions do not encourage a long stay.

There are two small social clubs, run by the occupational therapists, which meet weekly. These cater for about 50 patients each. There is also a social club on the neurosis unit, but this is scarcely a club, properly speaking, since it includes all patients, who take a hand in arranging their own activities.

Group Meetings

The medical superintendent's meetings with the consultants and with the whole medical staff have already been mentioned. The matron has a monthly meeting with the sisters, and the chief male nurse with charge nurses. At the patient-level, there are the meetings of the three social club committees. Communication at all these meetings tends to be one-way—*de haut en bas*—and there are no channels for the upwards movement of ideas, for broad discussions, or for the delegation of decision-making. Perhaps these things are not possible in so large a structure of such a composition; and the experience of the psychiatrist who tried to organize group therapy in the neurosis unit may be instructive on this point.

Briefly, he tried to reconstruct the social grouping of the unit by instituting an interrelated and carefully structured series of group meetings. These included a doctors' meeting, a senior staff meeting (doctors, sister, charge nurse, occupational therapy staff and social worker), a patients' committee, and a patients' general meeting. All these began with promise, ran for a few weeks, and then collapsed—apparently for different reasons.

The doctors' meeting collapsed because all four doctors attended on a sessional basis only, and it proved impossible to get them all there at the same time because of extra-mural commitments.

The senior staff meeting collapsed because the sister and the charge nurse were not receptive to new ideas. In meetings, they tended to take up a rigid attitude, and were unhelpful. They soon began to formulate excuses for not attending, and finally the meetings ceased.

The patients' committee was stopped because it apparently ran a great deal too well. It developed a group entity of its own which became set in opposition against the staff—as one doctor said, 'It was at us the whole time, agitating.'

The patients' general meeting collapsed because the doctors felt the verbalization level was too low for it to have any real value. A few patients from the patients' committee dominated it. The rest could not take any active part in it, and tended to sit passively.

The psychiatrist concerned thinks that the fundamental causes of failure were two-fold: the inability of nursing staff and patients to express themselves adequately in words, which led to hostility or passivity in different groups; and the lack of any real delegation of responsibility—'we just expected them to sit and talk'.

Lack of Communication

One of the major difficulties in carrying out research at Northtown was that there appeared to be no regular means of disseminating information. No Annual Report is issued, so that it is difficult to obtain information about who is employed by the hospital, what their work is, and what their qualifications are. It was often necessary to ask each person individually, since they did not know these facts about each other. Most members of staff were reasonably well-informed about members of their own professional group—provided that they worked in the same part of the hospital; and we formed a strong impression of a series of almost water-tight groups, working side by side, but making very little impact on one another. Doctors, nurses and administrators belong to large and well-organized professional groups, and do not feel a lack of communication, because they tend to think primarily within the professional orbit; but members of smaller groups and newer professions, such as the psychologists, the social workers, and others, are very dependent on co-operation with other groups, and do not always secure it. Some examples of lack of communication between groups are given below.

1. *The psychologists*, for example, are dependent on co-operation with the medical staff for the effectiveness of their work. Some psychiatrists regularly send patients to them for diagnostic tests, leaving them free to use what tests they think appropriate, and accepting their results as those of experts in their own field. Others specify the tests they wish to be used—and these may be out of date, because few psychiatrists keep up with the rapid developments made in psychological testing; and there are some who never send them patients, probably because they do not know quite what a psychologist does, and what help he can give. They never find out, because they never meet the psychologists in a professional setting. The psychologists are not invited to medical meetings, nor can they take their meals in the doctors' dining-room. They eat alone in their office, having refused to join a mess for junior O.T. staff on the grounds that this would imply a lowering of their professional status. Their social isolation reflects their professional isolation.

2. *The social workers* similarly cannot take a social history except on direct request from a psychiatrist. They find that some doctors use their services a great deal, and others not at all—depending largely on whether the individual doctor understands what a social worker is for, and what part she can play in caring for the patient. The question of status at meal-times arose with social workers too. During a period of reorganization, it was decided that they should share a dining-room with senior female nursing staff; and it was noticeable that this arrangement pleased neither side. Even when only one social worker and one assistant matron lunched at the same time, they ate at separate tables and barely acknowledged each other's existence. There was no personal animosity in this, and their professional relations were good. It was simply a mutual recognition of the fact that they belonged to different groups which erected an invisible wall between them.

3. *The senior tutor* in the Preliminary Training School is appointed by the Nursing Area Training Committee, and is allowed £75 per annum for the maintenance of furniture and the buying of equipment and films. This small sum is passed through the hospital accounts for administrative convenience, though it is granted by the Area Training Committee for use at the senior tutor's discretion. During the last year, he has asked that this sum should be devoted to the purchase of a tape-recorder for training purposes. This proposal has been vetoed—he is not sure by whom, or at what level.

4. *The catering officer* has tried to improve communication between the patients, the nursing staff and her own staff by sending out each week a sheet of menus with space for comments by nursing staff—either their own comments, or reported comments by patients—to be filled in daily on the meals served. If these were properly completed, they would provide her with knowledge of how the meals were received on the wards and help in future planning; but very few returns are adequately filled in. One or two sisters and charge nurses take the trouble to write helpful comments and criticisms. The rest simply write 'satisfactory' against each meal, day after day. There is no way of knowing whether this is fair comment or simply the quickest way out of what they feel to be simply another routine task; and there are too many sisters and charge nurses for the catering

officer to take the matter up personally with each, and to explain what she wants.

Anybody who visits a mental hospital and interviews staff can collect complaints. No group of people in a work-situation is likely to be entirely without malcontents, and no organization functions perfectly; but two points should be made clear. First, none of the information given above was phrased in the form of a complaint—it emerged spontaneously as members of staff talked about their work, its limitations and its possibilities. Second, wherever people felt a dissatisfaction with their role in the hospital—and there were other examples which we have no space to quote here—the factors involved pointed in the same direction: to a lack of communication between individuals and between groups. Probably the members of staff concerned have not arrived at this conclusion themselves—nobody phrased it in general terms, and each tends to think of his own problems, not of overall problems of policy.

Lack of communication is a problem inherent in any large-scale institution. The main group is so vast that it becomes ill-defined in the minds of those who work for it, and people tend to think in terms of 'my ward' or 'my profession' rather than of 'Northtown' as the centre of loyalty. The result is that the work of the hospital becomes fragmented, and some parts, particularly the smaller ones, do not work at full potential.

Patient Grouping

Patient groups must exist, and in so large a community, with so many long-stay patients, there must be many of a semi-permanent nature; but, with the exception of the two social club committees and the groupings in the neurosis unit, these do not appear to be known to the staff in general. Individual psychiatrists, sisters and charge nurses can describe in detail 'who makes friends with whom' on a particular ward; but this knowledge is not systematized or recognized as being of any importance to the hospital's main purpose. One is left with an impression of a staff-life and a patient-life existing side by side, but again without means of contact, except in fortuitous and individual cases; and these are a small minority.

Conclusion

Northtown is a hospital with many fundamental disadvantages. Its history, its architecture and above all its size, are all factors which weigh heavily against modern conceptions of care and treatment. The geographical division of the buildings adds to the difficulty of welding it into an integrated community, and the only solution to its inherent problems has been the concentration of authority in the hands of an energetic medical superintendent who virtually holds the scattered departments and buildings together as a unit by the strength of his own personality.

The medical staff is small, and, with notable exceptions, not highly trained; at the same time, the laboratory and technical services are very good. These factors taken in conjunction make it inevitable that the orientation of the hospital should be an organic one, physical methods of treatment being used in almost all cases.

Facilities and amenities which depend for their success on capital equipment operate at a high level of efficiency. What Northtown cannot do is to personalize those services for the individual patient.

IV

MOORDALE

MOORDALE was opened in 1900 as a hospital for private patients, run by a county authority. In 1948, it became a Health Service hospital, operating as part of a mixed group, and retaining a proportion of private and amenity beds.

The hospital thus has a mixed heritage, with some of the features of Crown Lodge, and some of Northtown. Like Crown Lodge, it is small (400 beds), and was designed for fee-paying patients. Like Northtown, it was founded by a county authority, and is now within the Health Service.

Moordale was originally chosen as the third hospital for the present survey in the hope that its combination of features of the other two hospitals would throw light on their problems and facilitate comparison. In fact, Moordale is in many ways different from both, and the administrative pattern is quite distinct. This outline of conditions at Moordale is therefore presented as an independent study.

Moordale's pre-Health Service status, as a private hospital run by a county authority, was unique. The motive for founding the hospital must have been similar to that which led to the foundation of Crown Lodge—a desire to make separate provision for middle-class patients who could pay a little towards the cost of treatment, because the general provisions for the mentally ill in that area were of a low standard. The eighteenth-century response to this idea was to set up a subscription hospital, independent of statutory control. The response at the end of the nineteenth century was to set up a hospital of similar type, but under the aegis of the county council. This was a period in which county and county borough councils were acquiring many new responsibilities.

There was a difference in operation. Crown Lodge was primarily a charitable institution, free to admit patients at less than the standard fee, or in special circumstances for no payment at all. Moordale, being subject to a degree of public accountability, could not do this. There was a set rate for 'in-county' patients, and another, slightly higher, for 'out-county' patients.

The medical superintendent at Moordale enjoyed a high degree of local autonomy. He was directly responsible to the county authority, and the fact that the hospital could accept patients from outside the county area gave it an almost national status. The hospital's position contrasted favourably with that of a neighbouring county asylum of the Northtown type. It was small, the buildings were pleasant and well equipped, the view was superb, and it attracted the 'better' staff and patients because of the amenities it had to offer.

When the Health Service came into operation, Moordale's position changed abruptly. The chief factors in the change were subordination to a Hospital Management Committee based elsewhere, loss of national and regional status, the substitution of a degree of lay administration for the unchallenged medical administration of former days, and (in the first few years of the Health Service) a comparative shortage of material resources.

The decision to incorporate Moordale into a group of hospitals based elsewhere was due to a number of considerations. First, the hospital was considered too small to form a reasonable administrative unit on its own. The expense of carrying out accounting, dispensing or supplies separately for such a small unit might have been disproportionate.[1] Secondly, the policy of the Region was to integrate general hospitals and mental hospitals at group level where possible. Only two Regional Hospital Boards pursued this policy. (Others preferred to create separate 'mental groups', maintaining that the needs and administrative traditions of mental hospitals were quite

[1] On the other hand, the World Health Organization's Expert Committee on Mental Health (3rd Report, 1953) states, p. 29: 'From the point of view of financial economy, the optimum capacity for hospitals probably lies between 250 and 400 beds.'

distinct, and could not be merged at group level with those of general hospitals.) In Moordale's region, the aim was to design each group in such a way that it would cover the varied hospital needs, including psychiatric needs, of a given area. On the Appointed Day, therefore, the hospital ceased to be autonomous, and became part of a group which also includes a general hospital, a convalescent hospital, a maternity hospital, and a children's hospital. Group headquarters is situated at the general hospital, three miles from Moordale.

This involved some decrease in status. Instead of being in a distinct and separate relationship with the county authority, Moordale is now one of a number of hospitals in a group centred elsewhere.

Loss of national and regional status has also resulted from changes in the patient-population. On the Appointed Day, the old distinction between 'in-county' and 'out-county' patients was abolished, and three types of patients were admitted: Health Service patients (section 3) were to be admitted from a small local catchment area, and were limited to 20 per cent of available beds. Amenity patients (section 4) might be admitted from anywhere in the Regional Board area, and were allotted 60 per cent of beds. Private patients (section 5) might, as before, be admitted without restrictions as to place of residence, and were allotted 20 per cent of beds.

Since 1948, the cost of section 4 and section 5 beds has increased sharply. The weekly fee for private patients was then 3½–4½ guineas per week, and is now 10 guineas. That for amenity patients was thirty-five shillings for a single room, and is now 4 guineas. In the interval, the National Health Service has become generally accepted, and the middle classes no longer

TABLE 3

Allocation of beds at Moordale

	Percentage of total beds	
	July 1948*	July 1958†
Health Service	20·0	41·7
Amenity	60·0	43·7
Private	20·0	14·6

* Proportions as laid down on the Appointed Day.
† Actual bed-occupation to one decimal point.

have much money to spare for preferential treatment in times of illness. Consequently, the proportions have changed. Health Service patients have increased in numbers, while private and amenity patients have decreased (see Table 3, p. 83).

These figures indicate a progressive restriction in the hospital's sphere of influence. As the number of Health Service patients rises, Moordale becomes increasingly a local hospital with a catchment area rather than a hospital with national and regional status.

The decline in medical administration results from incorporation into a mixed hospital group. The chief officer of the group is the group secretary, a lay administrator; and although the position of medical superintendents of mental hospitals was specifically safeguarded by regulation in 1948,[1] the superimposition of group organization meant a diminution in responsibility for the medical superintendent at Moordale, and an increased degree of lay administration. The implications of this change will be discussed later.

The comparative shortage of material resources was again due to incorporation into a hospital group. In the first few years of the Health Service, there was much to be done in order to bring all hospitals up to the new standards. Unlike most mental hospitals, Moordale had enjoyed a favoured position and was comparatively well equipped. The financial resources of the group were naturally concentrated on the less-favoured hospitals in the interim period of reorganization.

Moordale's immediate background is therefore one of decline in prestige and responsibility. A hospital which was once of national status is in the process of being assimilated into the Health Service pattern. Initially this meant levelling-down rather than levelling-up—a somewhat painful process of readjustment.

Site, Buildings, and Distribution of Patients

The hospital is situated in a rural area, on the edge of a small

[1] S.I. 1948 No. 419, which states: 'The Superintendent shall be the chief officer of the hospital . . . and he shall be responsible for the general management thereof in accordance with any directions which may be given by the Regional Hospital Board or the Hospital Management Committee. . . .' This was rescinded in 1960 (after the survey at Moordale had taken place), though the contractual rights of medical superintendents then in office were safeguarded.

village. Group headquarters is three miles away, in a market town. The nearest large industrial centre, where the Region's university is situated, is fifteen miles away.

Moordale consists of a main block for male and female patients, two small villas, and a private house, 'The Mount', which is used as a half-way house for women patients soon to be discharged. It is surrounded by well-kept gardens and extensive grounds in a setting of sweeping hills and valleys, as yet untouched by industry or housing projects.

The state of decoration, furnishing and repair in the main building speaks eloquently of the hospital's past history and present policy. There is the basic, solid Edwardian structure, and a good deal of solid Edwardian equipment and furniture which was of excellent quality in its day but is now due for replacement. There is clear evidence of a gap in provision—of furnishings grown shabby, of wards repainted by unskilled hands, of flimsy coverings and curtains. This represents the war period, when new materials and skilled labour were not available, and the early Health Service period, when group resources were mainly concentrated on the other hospitals. There is also evidence of a change in policy in the last three or four years—good new furniture, expert re-decoration, new fireplaces and light fitments and good quality curtains and covers. Present policy can be deduced from the fact that these new resources have been spread throughout the hospital, long-stay and short-stay wards alike, rather than being concentrated on the 'shop window' of short-stay care. For example, Vynide-covered chairs have been provided in the sitting-rooms for the more deteriorated patients. These are easily sponged, and no patient now has to be kept in bed purely because of incontinence. Some wards have new curtains, others new chairs, and others new carpets. None has yet been completely re-furnished, so that the effect is diffused; but this may be preferable to some very well equipped wards and some still in a pre-war condition.

There are four wards for male patients, and four for female patients. On each side, ward 1 is the admission and treatment ward, ward 2 for better short-stay patients, ward 3 (closed) for deteriorated or demented patients, and ward 4 for stabilized long-stay patients. The number of patients on a ward varies from 29 to 50.

Internal architecture is more formalized than at Crown Lodge, but much less so than at Northtown. Each ward has an outer door, and is approached via a separate staircase or corridor; but within the ward, arrangements are informal. There are many single rooms, and each ward has two or more sitting-rooms, a dining-room and several small dormitory-bedrooms, none of which takes more than 12 patients. There are alcoves and odd corners where patients can sit in small groups. Sitting-rooms and alcoves are left to natural cliquing.

Wards M3 and F3 are the only closed wards in the hospital. They contain 73 patients in all—about 17 per cent of the total patient-population.

The two villas are modern and well furnished. They take a mixture of short-stay patients in the convalescent stage, and long-stay patients who have reached a fairly high degree of socialization. Again, natural cliquing plays a part; for some patients ask to be transferred to a villa so that they can be with their friends, while others prefer to stay in the main building. In a small hospital, rigid classification by diagnosis or symptomatology is not possible, and at Moordale it has not been attempted. Some patients have to stay on certain wards because of the need for observation or treatment. Others can exercise a certain degree of choice.

'The Mount' is a large house, still furnished as a house, and not as a hospital annexe. From 12 to 15 women are accommodated there, under the supervision of a sympathetic sister of domestic inclinations. Groups of three or four take it in turns to clean, cook, and carry out other normal household duties. Food supplies are sent over from the main kitchens. The patients decide on their own menus, and prepare the food in a large, homely kitchen with an Aga cooker. A period of a month or six weeks at 'The Mount' is intended as a re-introduction to domestic responsibilities and home life immediately prior to discharge from hospital.

The administrative officers are at the centre of the main block, with the exception of the lay administrative offices, which are at the back of the hospital, near the laundry and the kitchens. The matron and the chief male nurse each have an office, in the female wing and the male wing respectively.

Behind the main administrative offices lies the 'social centre'

—the hall, the canteen, and a stretch of wide corridor banked with potted plants and flowers. This last area stretches for perhaps fifty yards from the entrance to the male wing to the entrance to the female wing, and contains several long seats, two telephone kiosks, a stamp machine, a cigarette machine, and a variety of notice-boards bearing information about hospital events. What might be a characterless stretch of hospital corridor has been given something of the atmosphere of a village square.

The hall is equipped with a stage and a piano, and a moveable pitch-pine pulpit for Sunday services (there is no separate Church). The canteen is open every day from 10 a.m. to 4 p.m., sells a wide variety of goods, and provides hot drinks and snacks, with seating accommodation for 20 or 30 patients. The library contains about 500 books belonging to the hospital on open shelves, and a small case from the County Library which is changed every month. The latter is kept locked, and opened only at certain hours rare enough to be listed on the Entertainments programme.

All wards have television sets: in all but the sick wards, these are placed in the dining-rooms, so that the slight deterrent of sitting on a hard chair shall induce patients to seek more profitable forms of activity. Television is meant to be an occasional relaxation, not a means of 'keeping the patients quiet'.

Administration

Before 1948, administration at Moordale was centralized, the medical superintendent having full executive control. Since then, the position has changed considerably.

The Hospital Management Committee sits at group headquarters. There is a small House Committee for Moordale, but all decisions must be ratified by the main committee. The House Committee represents the Group's interest at Moordale rather than representing Moordale's interest at Group.

No other hospital in the group has a medical superintendent, and in each the hospital secretary is the chief administrative officer. The chain of command runs smoothly from hospital secretaries to group secretary. All are lay administrators, with similar qualifications (A.H.A. or F.H.A.), a common professional affiliation (to the Institute of Hospital Administrators), common values, assumptions, and attitudes. At Moordale, and only at Moordale, the chief administrator is a psychiatrist. His qualifications are medical ones, his professional affiliation is to the British Medical Association and the Royal Medico-Psychological Association, his values, attitudes and assumptions have been formed in a different environment. To all the basic differences between a general hospital and a mental hospital are added differences between a lay administrator who has 'come up through the office' with experience of supplies and finance, and a psychiatrist, who has spent most of his working life on the wards and in the clinics.

This leads to a potentially difficult situation between group secretary, hospital secretary, and medical superintendent. The group secretary tends to use the same channels of communication at Moordale as at the other hospitals, particularly in dealing with matters which concern all of them. It is easier to treat all hospital secretaries alike—particularly for a man who was once a hospital secretary himself.

The medical superintendent may appreciate this position but is scarcely likely to condone it. He was already in office in 1948, so that he administered Moordale in the days when there was no appreciable lay intervention. He is conscious that there is also a strong 'anti-superintendent' movement within the medical profession; and that before he reaches retiring age he may be regarded simply as one consultant among several.

The hospital secretary has the difficulty of serving two masters—for there is no clear line of demarcation between those matters for which he is responsible to the medical superintendent, and those for which he is directly responsible to the group secretary.

Thus the position is a difficult one for all three. The group secretary is aware that he does not have quite the same degree of control over Moordale as over his other hospitals. The medical superintendent is aware that his position is not what it was before 1948. The hospital secretary is aware that his responsibility and prestige are less than those of other hospital secretaries in the same group. The three-cornered structure involves a general dispersal of authority.

This is a built-in problem, inherent in the organization of a mixed group containing a mental hospital—and not, of course, peculiar to Moordale, since there are other mental hospitals which work in a similar framework. It exists independently of personal and temperamental factors; and perhaps it should be said that the people who hold these offices in Moordale's group work together at present with a degree of harmony which is in general a tribute to their administrative ability. Nevertheless, the situation can produce difficulties; and four illustrations of the way in which it affects departmental work are given below:

1. *The Catering Officer* is responsible for drawing up menus and preparing food. He is responsible in theory to the medical superintendent for the quality of food served to patients and staff; but marketing is handled by the lay administrative staff. There is a group farm, which once belonged to Moordale. Produce from the farm is now allocated among the hospitals in the group by headquarters staff. The catering officer has to accept his share, whether this is what he wishes to order or not, and it is costed at open market prices. At one time, he was sent £50 worth of milk weekly surplus to his requirements. This had to be used or thrown away. In the winter, he is frequently supplied with prime English meat when much cheaper imported meat would make excellent stews, puddings and pies.

For items of foodstuff other than those supplied from the farms and gardens, he prepares marketing lists, which he hands to the hospital secretary, who in turn passes them to the group secretary. These lists are subject to alteration at hospital or group level, without prior consultation or subsequent notification. The catering officer submits his lists. In due course, he receives his supplies, less any items vetoed by his unseen mentors. He does not know the name or official position of the person who actually handles his lists at Group; and he cannot talk to him, since he has no telephone.

2. *Gardens*. The head gardener at Moordale is responsible directly to the group secretary, and through him to the Farms and Gardens sub-committee. This sub-committee controls all the garden-work in the group, and the primary aim is to provide fresh, cheap produce. At Moordale, and at no other

hospital in the group, patients work in the gardens. The Farm and Gardens sub-committee tend to regard patient labour as 'inefficient'. The medical superintendent and medical staff regard it as a therapeutic activity in which the end-product is comparatively unimportant. To them the head gardener is primarily a person who is in charge of groups of patients rather than a person who produces flowers and vegetables. The head gardener is thus subject to contradictory pressures from the staff at Moordale, with whom he comes into daily contact, and the staff and management committee at Group, to whom he is responsible.

3. *The occupational therapists* are responsible to the medical superintendent, but the supply of materials for occupational therapy is a matter for the lay administrative staff. Some materials used in occupational therapy work can only be ordered from one particular firm; but the routine practice of inviting tenders from three firms is still followed—even though two will regularly reply that they do not stock the item. This involves unnecessary work and expense.

The occupational therapy department is expected to buy in bulk twice a year, though materials get soiled and crushed, and storage space is very limited.

4. *The clinical secretaries* work directly with the medical staff, but are regarded as part of the hospital secretary's department. If they work overtime, as they often do, since they are short-staffed, it is at the request of one of the doctors. If they ask for time off in lieu, the request must go to the secretary's office—and may well be denied on the grounds that other lay administrative staff do not have time off in working hours. There is a general lack of communication between the medical staff and the lay administrative staff—typified by the fact that the clinical offices are at the front of the hospital, and the lay administrative offices at the back.

In a number of departments, a dichotomy is felt between the interests of Group and the interests of Moordale. Group is identified with general hospital interests and lay administration; Moordale, with mental hospital interests and medical administration. There is a strong feeling in some quarters that Moordale has been 'occupied territory' since 1948; and this shows no sign of decreasing.

Group Structure at Moordale

Despite—or possibly because of—the problems inherent in the hospital's relations with the group, relations between departments and between staff and patients are generally very good. In the government of a country, home affairs are generally easier to manage when foreign policy is difficult—and the same may be true for a hospital, the existence of external problems furthering internal cohesion.

There are four formal groups which meet regularly, and which are described below. The nature of semi-formal and informal groupings will be indicated subsequently.

(*a*) *The Staff Meeting and 'Monday Round'* (weekly). The Staff Meeting takes place at 9 a.m. on Mondays, and consists in effect of a review of the past week's work and a discussion of plans for the week to come. The medical superintendent takes the chair. The meeting is attended by all medical staff, the hospital secretary, the matron and chief male nurse, the psychiatric social worker, and one of the social therapists.

The head gardener attends for a few minutes at the beginning of the meeting—a reminder that his work has a therapeutic element, and perhaps a reflection of the conflict in policy with regard to the gardens which has already been noted. After giving a report on the activities of patient working-parties, he withdraws. The rest of the meeting, which lasts one hour, is taken up with discussion of general administrative matters and of policy with regard to individual patients. There are short case-discussions to which various members of staff present will contribute from their own knowledge of the patient before a decision (e.g. to try a new treatment, to discharge, or to interview relatives) is made.

At 10 o'clock, the secretary and the social therapist withdraw, and the meeting resolves itself into the 'Monday Round'. Headed by the medical superintendent, the group visits every ward, talking to staff and patients. The matron withdraws while the male side is visited, and the chief male nurse withdraws while the female side is visited; otherwise, the group remains intact until the round ends at approximately 1.30 p.m.

Most contacts are brief, but the medical superintendent will pause from time to time to discuss an unusual clinical problem with the medical staff, to consult the doctor responsible where a patient makes a request, to bring the psychiatric social worker into a case where she may be needed, or simply to talk for some time to a patient who is worried or distressed. Sometimes the group will split up on a ward, various members talking to nursing staff or patients.

Although the round lasts for three and a half hours, it is not possible to do justice in this time to all wards. To ensure that no ward is overlooked or hastily dealt with, the round begins on the male side and the female side in alternate weeks. The side which is visited first is dealt with thoroughly and at leisure, the other side more speedily.

The 'Monday Round' has obvious similarities to a consultant's clinical round in a teaching hospital, and this is typical of medical policy at Moordale. Of the four major group meetings, three have a teaching purpose. The medical superintendent is also Lecturer in Psychiatry in the Region's university;[1] and the younger members of his staff are studying for the Diploma in Psychological Medicine. Moordale has many of the features of a post-graduate teaching hospital, though it is not formally recognized as such.

The round brings the doctors in touch with all wards and all patients. This is valuable, particularly for young doctors, who might otherwise be assigned to one or two wards and have a limited knowledge of the rest of the hospital. It helps the medical staff in discussing their patients with one another, since they all have some personal contact with the patient under discussion. It enables all patients to be seen, and their problems to be dealt with at the highest level. Any patient can approach the medical superintendent with complaints or requests, without difficulty, and without intermediaries. The round also keeps a high standard on the wards, since visitation by a group of eight or nine people at once can be very thorough.

There are some disadvantages. The round is time-consuming, and all members of staff involved are absent from their normal duties for the whole of a long and often exhausting morning. It seems to create tensions in some patients. Some try to keep

[1] The medical superintendent at Crown Lodge holds a similar title, but has no regular teaching responsibilities in the university Department of Psychiatry for that Region.

out of the way until it has passed, lingering in wash-rooms and lavatories. Some spend half the morning rehearsing what they are going to say, and then are too shy or too tense to speak up in the face of such a gathering; and the occasional exhibitionist tends to take advantage of the situation, though the staff can generally discriminate between those who need attention and those who merely like it.

(*b*) *The Medical Clinical Meeting* (weekly). This meeting is attended by all medical staff, the psychiatric social worker, and psychiatrists from neighbouring hospitals. Members of the medical staff take it in turn to read a paper, usually presenting a case for clinical discussion. A patient may be asked to attend and to answer questions from those present. The meeting provides a forum for psychiatric discussion, a means by which the individual psychiatrist can get a wider view, and the opinions of his colleagues, on a difficult case.

Patients who had attended such meetings were interviewed during the course of the survey. All said that they had been treated with courtesy, and that they were flattered to feel that their problems were receiving so much expert attention. They seemed to find little stress in attending the meetings, and often actually enjoyed them.

(*c*) *The Nurses' Clinical Meeting* (weekly) is run on similar lines. Again, the medical superintendent takes the chair. The meeting is attended by some senior nursing staff; by the psychiatric social worker; by the student nurses, for whom this is part of the course for the Mental Nursing Certificate; and by local authority mental welfare officers, who come by invitation when they can. The medical staff take it in turns to act as tutor to the group, giving a paper on some aspect of clinical psychiatry. The student nurses thus have a variety of lecturers, and get to know the doctors. Senior nurses are able to refresh their knowledge. Local authority staff make contact with nursing and medical staff, and learn a little psychiatry. The medical staff are given experience in teaching—quite a difficult assignment in this case, since it is necessary to provide material which is sufficiently advanced to interest the senior staff present, while yet being intelligible to student nurses.

Since the full-time medical staff is only six in number, the practice of having a paper read at both the Medical Clinical

Meeting and the Nurses' Clinical Meeting weekly means that every doctor, from the medical superintendent down to the junior house medical officers, has to prepare and deliver a paper on an average once every three weeks.

(*d*) *The Patients' Social Club Meeting* (weekly) is presided over by one of the medical staff, who takes the chair by personal invitation from the ward representatives. The psychiatric social worker and one of the social therapists attend. Discussion is primarily centred on plans concerning patients' entertainments—games, tournaments, ward parties, films, outside trips, and so on. The ward representatives may also raise points connected with welfare and ward organization. The doctor who takes the chair may deal with these points in discussion; or, if he thinks that action should be taken, he will refer them directly to the medical superintendent, or bring them up at the Staff Meeting on the following Monday.

(*e*) *Semi-formal and informal groups* are numerous. They take many forms, and are usually of an ad hoc nature, so that it is difficult to classify them. A doctor or senior nurse will call a ward together for discussion of an issue of general interest. A doctor may start group therapy sessions on a particular ward because he is interested in group dynamics, and feels that a certain group of patients would profit from this approach. A group of staff, or patients, or patients and staff combined, may find common interests in music or drama, and arrange to meet for gramophone recitals, or to produce a play. The social therapists, whose work is described later, do much to foster such interests, and groups often form round them.

This activity is qualitatively different from the 'therapeutic community' system, as practised at Crown Lodge. Moordale groups meet for a teaching purpose, or to discuss certain issues for their own sake, or for some activity. Human relationships may improve in the process, but this improvement is a by-product rather than the main purpose.

The Medical Staff

There are six full-time doctors: the medical superintendent; a consultant, who acts in the medical superintendent's place when he is absent but who is not designated as deputy medical superintendent; a senior hospital medical officer; a senior registrar; a registrar, and one junior house medical officer. The first three hold the Diploma in Psychological Medicine, and the last three are working for it. Junior staff have a regular 'study day' weekly, which they spend in the university Department of Psychiatry, either at lectures or in the library.

The consultant is secretary of a regional psychiatric association, to which all members of the medical staff, the psychiatric social worker, and some of the nursing staff belong. The association admits psychiatrists and other medical practitioners as full members, and other workers connected with mental health work as associate members. Monthly meetings and occasional social events are held.

The medical superintendent, consultant and senior house medical officer are responsible for out-patient clinics in neighbouring towns.

These activities, together with the time spent on teaching groups and the Monday Round, improve the quality of clinical work in the hospital, and increase its psychiatric influence (i.e. influence on doctors, social workers and patients, as distinct from prestige with the general public) in the Region. At the same time, they inevitably curtail the amount of time which the small medical staff can devote to their present patients. The average amount of clinical time devoted to each patient was 35·0 minutes per week for short-stay patients, and 13·7 minutes per week for long-stay patients.

To an observer, the most striking factor about the medical staff at Moordale is their variety of outlook. There is no one dominant school of psychiatric thought. The atmosphere is an academic one, in which all schools of thought are considered, each doctor contributes what he can to discussion from his own experience and reading, and there is a genuine spirit of enquiry.

There is an up-to-date medical library, which is in frequent use.

Nursing Staff

The total nursing staff is 119½ (part-timers equated to full-timers) plus 18 nursing cadets. Full establishment is 121, so there is no appreciable shortage; but the matron and the chief male nurse point out that they have 'the wrong assortment'. There are only four staff nurses, though the establishment is for 17; and the shortage of trained nursing staff has been made up with untrained nursing assistants.

There are a few staff houses, but these are in the village, not on a hospital estate. Most of the nursing staff live in the village, and there appears to be little feeling either for or against hospital houses. Quarters for resident female nursing staff are provided in a large converted house near the hospital; male nursing staff have rather cramped quarters in the hospital itself.

The chief male nurse mentioned the shortage of trained mental nurses, but said that he was able to exercise a good deal of selection among applicants for junior nursing posts. Those he rejected often went to the big mental hospital near by:

There they get into the big institutional method of nursing. They shout and bully. . . . Where you get one nurse with a little group of patients, he's got to get on with them.

Both male and female nurses work the 'short day': day shifts from 6 a.m. to 2 p.m., and 2 p.m. to 10 p.m., with a night shift from 10 p.m. to 6 a.m. A scheme for a 44-hour week (or rather, an 88-hour fortnight, since it is not possible to arrange hours more exactly with a relatively small staff) has been prepared, and will be put into effect as soon as the other hospitals in the group are ready to do the same.

Male nurses and female nurses seem to work well together on the whole. The male nurses, as at the other hospitals, complain that mental nursing is under feminine domination; but criticism centres not on the female nurses at Moordale, but on the Royal College of Nursing:

'They won't accept that it (mental nursing) has ceased to be a vocation—it's a man's bread and butter now.'

'They don't give mental nursing a fair deal—they look down on us for some reason, especially the men.'

'All those old matrons . . .'

This seems to be a fairly superficial type of grumbling, due to a feeling of lack of prestige in comparison to nurses at general hospitals. There are apparently no specific causes of discontent, and trade union activity is virtually non-existent.

The secretary of the Confederation of Health Service Employees is a male nurse. He used to call meetings regularly each month, but no one attended, and so he ceased to do so. Some notices on the C.O.H.S.E. notice-board are two years old.

There is no chairman or treasurer, and the secretary doubts whether he has a constitutional right to hold office, since there have been no elections for three years. He collects Union subscriptions, which are sent on to headquarters less his own commission; but he says, 'There's no need for a Union here. We might as well pay our four shillings a week to the Staff Social Club.'

'If we have any problems, I can always see the chief male nurse or the medical superintendent. It's easier to get things done on the spot—there's no need to involve outsiders. The staff are almost mollycoddled here—the medical superintendent asks how they are getting on, encourages them to pass exams, and lends them his own books . . .'

The secretary of C.O.H.S.E. is subject to conflicting pressures. On one hand, as a trade union organizer, he would like to have a strong branch, and causes in which to lead his members. On the other, he is honest enough to admit that there are no causes, and that the need simply does not arise. His use of the term 'outsiders' in speaking of his own Union officials indicates that his loyalty is primarily to the hospital, not to the Union.

There is no N.U.P.E. organization at Moordale. Lay administrative staff belong to N.A.L.G.O., which is organized from group headquarters.

Ancillary Departments

Dispensing is carried out from a central dispensary at group headquarters. Each ward sends over a daily order, countersigned by the psychiatrist in charge. It is not easy to get drugs at short notice, other than at the regular times, from group headquarters. As a result, the male and female admission and treatment wards (M1 and F1) indulge in unofficial stockpiling, and other wards draw on them for small supplies when these are needed urgently. The group dispensary is efficient and well organized; but in view of its distance from Moordale, stock-piling on a small scale is probably inevitable. The effect is to place some drug supplies under the control of the nursing staff, not the medical staff. However, we found that drug books were kept punctiliously, and could find no suggestion of laxity in administration.

Records. The records room is very small, and usually crowded, as medical staff and clinical secretaries come in to consult case-papers. Records are kept efficiently, and cross-indexed. As at Crown Lodge, staff can often recall details about a given patient without reference to the case-papers; and their interest appears to go on long after patients are discharged. During the follow-up study, we found many odd notes on patients' subsequent progress in their files. These had been contributed by doctors at out-patient clinics, by local authority workers, and in one or two instances by members of the nursing staff. Records are shortly to be decentralized, since the accommodation is very cramped. Those for patients in the hospital will be kept on the wards, where they will be more easily accessible to the medical staff concerned. The records room will then deal only with records of patients who have been discharged.

The Social Worker. There is one fully-trained psychiatric social worker. The degree to which she is integrated in the work of the hospital has already been indicated—she takes part in the Staff Meeting, accompanies the medical staff on the Monday Round, attends the Nurses' Clinical Meeting and the Patients' Social Club Meeting. She is fully part of the team, not simply someone to whom case-work problems can be referred. She works closely with the medical staff. She carries out domiciliary visits, mainly to the relatives of patients who are in hospital or to patients who are about to be admitted; but the relationship with local authority Mental Health Departments is a flexible one, and she sometimes follows up patients, keeping in touch with local authority workers.

Liaison with local authority mental welfare officers is excellent. They have a standing invitation to the Nurses' Clinical Meeting, and those who come usually visit the psychiatric worker's office on the same morning, discussing their cases and general problems. In many ways the psychiatric social worker acts almost in a consultative capacity. She is well known in the area, belongs to the regional psychiatric association, and has taken part in organizing short courses for mental welfare officers arranged by the university Extra-Mural Department.

Her case-load is a fairly heavy one. In the first six months of 1958, she referred 90 cases to other agencies, and carried 74 herself. Of these cases, the overwhelming majority were concerned with personal and emotional problems rather than financial and material needs. A breakdown is given below:

TABLE 4

Social Case-work at Moordale, January–June 1958

(*a*) Referred cases:	
Financial or other material needs involved	19 cases
Financial, etc. needs not involved	71
	90
(*b*) P.S.W's own case-load:	
Financial or other material needs involved	17
Financial, etc. needs not involved	57
	74

Occupational Therapy. Accommodation for occupational therapy is also very cramped. A new O.T. unit was planned in 1939, but was not built, due to the shortage of resources during the war and in the early Health Service days. The project has now been revived, and it is hoped that the new centre will be started shortly. At present, occupational therapy for women takes place in two rooms, one of which is also a dining-room and has to be cleared for lunch. Occupational therapy for men takes place in a semi-basement, which again is not ideal for this purpose. One patient described it rather unjustly as 'a sinister cellar'.

About 40 patients of each sex attend occupational therapy at any one time. There are morning and afternoon shifts, so that roughly 160 patients are able to attend occupational therapy for half-days.

Traditional occupational therapy crafts—rug-making, basket-work, weaving, and so on—are pursued. There is no paid employment for patients apart from a little utility work.

Social Therapy. Moordale employs five social therapists.

Although one or two other mental hospitals also have workers with this title, there is no recognized training in social therapy, and no agreement as to the limitations and possibilities of the work as yet, so that the situation at Moordale is peculiar to that hospital.

The social therapists are all married women. They organize a wide variety of patients' activities, including gardening, play-reading, musical appreciation groups, tennis, bridge and whist, dancing classes, a choir, and physical training classes. They take patients shopping, arrange a programme of outside entertainments, organize coach outings, and run the small library. At Christmas, they produce a Nativity Play and arrange a Fancy Dress Ball, helping patients to obtain materials and to make their own costumes.

Among their regular weekly activities is a party for deteriorated long-stay patients. These are the patients who in some hospitals are regarded as 'hopeless'. To produce some degree of animation, even for a short time, is a difficult and superficially unrewarding task. The social therapists arrange a medley of dancing, community singing and musical solos in which no patient is overlooked, and all are encouraged to contribute a little, even if only by singing the chorus of a popular song. (Since this is a fairly elderly grouping, the most popular songs are those of 1914–18.) The important factor is that every patient present is made to feel that he (or she) matters, and that the party would be less of a sucess without him.

The work of the social therapists is an integral part of the hospital's programme. They work well in co-operation with the medical staff, but experience some difficulty with female nursing staff. Some senior nurses feel that the modern concept of psychiatric nursing includes the kind of activities which the social therapists undertake. One senior member of the nursing staff said:

> 'I very much disagree with all this social therapy business. It takes all the plum jobs away from the nurses, things they like doing, and just leaves them to guard the ward. It's considered all right for nurses to do things like scrubbing the floors, and these social therapists do all the valuable things. . . .'

Another thought that the resentment arose largely through

the social therapists' lack of settled status. They have no qualifications, and no professional organization; and it is widely known that they are paid at assistant nurses' rates. She pointed out that if they were 'experts' with a higher salary, their work might be treated with more respect.

It would be difficult for this work to be done by assistant nurses. The social therapists must be free to move round the hospital, and to consult all grades of staff in a way which would be impossible for a junior nurse. In this small hospital, they appear to fill a considerable need at a very low cost.

Patient Groupings

Patients at Moordale seem relatively free from community pressures—neither the therapeutically-designed pressures of Crown Lodge nor the institutional pressures of Northtown find a counterpart here. There are many facilities for patient activities and patient groups, but these form and change spontaneously; and staff often take part in them. There is not one level of 'staff life' and another of 'patient life'. The two interact and overlap.

At a Social Club Committee Meeting, ward representatives were asked to comment on the hospital, and on their own experiences:

MR. PRESTON: There's a swing away from the clinical approach, isn't there? That's certainly true here. You get small groups of patients and nurses together, not huge masses. Sort of gives the patient's personality a chance.

MR. PIPER: I think the approach is very good here. The doctors always listen to you. If you want to get hold of a doctor quickly, and he's busy, he'll leave a personal message for you. That's the kind of thing that counts.

In 'The Mount', the approach is rather different. This is a therapeutically-designed setting for a small and specific group. Here, women patients find a very strong group support in the difficult and often bewildering final stages of rehabilitation.

MISS PAXTON: When you come in here, you start at the back end. Everyone else is better than you are; but the people who are better pull you through.

MISS PERRYMAN: I've only just come, and I find it all a bit worrying.

MRS. PENROSE: Well, Miss Perryman, you've never done any cooking or housekeeping before, you see. Don't worry—there are always several of us on together, and the others will help.

Another patient at 'The Mount' commented on the role of the nursing sister in charge:

'It's more like a home than a hospital. Sister doesn't wear uniform in the afternoons—she comes in and talks to us, and does some knitting or sewing.'

Such permissiveness and informality are characteristic of staff-patient relationships at Moordale.

The Hospital and the Community

We have seen that Moordale is well based in its local community. The medical staff have close links with the university; the psychiatric social worker works in liaison with social workers in the area; psychiatrists, social worker and a number of nursing staff belong to the regional psychiatric association, which brings them into touch with staff from other mental hospitals, and from the university Department of Psychiatry. As at other hospitals within the Health Service, the medical staff also take out-patient clinics, and fulfil other advisory and consultant roles where necessary.

Relatives are welcome at Moordale. Visiting takes place on three afternoons a week, and in addition relatives may call for patients and take them out on any evening. Relatives get to know the nursing staff—and can sometimes be seen, on visiting days, not merely accepting a cup of tea from sister, but wandering round the small ward kitchen, helping to make it. Sometimes children are brought in—a rare feature in mental hospitals, and a tribute to Moordale's homely, pleasant atmosphere.

Like Crown Lodge, Moordale receives a fair number of alcoholics among its patients. Close contact is maintained with Alcoholics Anonymous. There is a strong and active branch of this organization in the nearby market town, and the present secretary is himself an ex-patient. His own addiction to alcohol was cured by treatment at Moordale followed by community help from A.A., and he is now doing what he can to help other patients, visiting them in hospital, and taking them out to group meetings.

Further links with the community result from the activities of the hospital's League of Friends. This group was formed six years ago on the initiative of the Hospital Management Committee, and the medical superintendent. The chairman is a member of the Management Committee, and herself a trained nurse.

There is no permanent and distinct membership of the group, apart from that of the committee of seven, all women, some of whom were originally invited to serve, and some of whom have been co-opted. Each committee member represents some local interest, such as the Mothers' Union, or the Women's Institute, and these organizations are asked to help the hospital in various ways.

The League of Friends has raised over £1,000 in its six years of operation, in addition to £350 which is specially earmarked for the equipment of a hospital Chapel. Money is raised by social events—a coffee morning or a small dance, an annual garden party and Christmas Fair—and has been spent on a variety of amenities for the patients. Among other items, a cricket pavilion has been provided, and a radiogram has recently been presented to 'The Mount'.

In addition to money-raising efforts, the League of Friends befriends individual patients. Lonely patients are visited, and sent individual Christmas presents. Patients are asked to tea in private homes, and taken for outings. Efforts are made to encourage other organizations to 'adopt' friendless long-stay patients, and to keep in permanent contact with them.

The form of organization—a self-perpetuating committee with no membership—is unusual, but quite workable in a village, where each committee member is recognized in her own right as one of the leaders of the community; and it means in effect a two-tier organization, since committee members can call on their own organizations for help, rather than starting a separate group.

Moordale's present position shows conflicting trends. Since

the Health Service came into operation, its prestige as a privileged hospital for well-to-do patients has declined. As far as this hospital at least is concerned, the Regional Board's policy of integrating mental and general hospitals in mixed groups has not been a success. It has resulted in administrative problems which are sometimes acute, and the adjustments involved have been difficult.

Yet Moordale's prestige in the purely psychiatric field is probably higher than it has ever been. Liaison and co-operation with community services, both statutory and voluntary, with other mental hospitals, and with the university, are very good.

Because this is a small hospital, it could not stand alone in the Health Service, providing all its own facilities. It had to rely to some extent on the facilities of the nearby general hospital, and a joint group organization was thus considered necessary. Because it is a small hospital, and perhaps because it is in some ways threatened by group organization, it is exceptionally united. It has few internal problems, and is able to play an active role in the life of the surrounding community.

PART THREE

Measures of Efficiency

V

NEEDS AND RESOURCES

Any comparison demands a base-line for reference. We cannot compare things which are totally unlike. A comparison in efficiency presents special difficulty, because it demands two base-lines. In order to compare the ways in which organizations are run, we have first to show that their needs are comparable, and then show that the resources which they bring to bear on them are comparable also.

Our studies of the administration of Crown Lodge, Northtown and Moordale show that they exhibit major differences in both needs and resources. In this chapter, we examine and summarize some of these differences, before proceeding to consider how far, and on what criteria, comparisons of efficiency can be made.

Organizational Aims

To say that the purpose of a mental hospital is 'to treat mental patients' is an over-simplification. We need to know what types of patients are treated; what are the aims of treatment; and whether there are any other legitimate aims of mental hospital organization.

(*a*) *Patient-populations*. It is sometimes assumed that patients in one mental hospital are very like patients in another. The phrase 'mental hospital patients' brings a stereotyped image to the mind; but it seemed probable that hospitals of such differing types would attract different types of patients. Analysis of the patient-population in the hospitals at the time of the survey

TABLE 5

Patient-census

	Percentage of standing population		
	Crown Lodge	Northtown	Moordale
1. SEX			
Male	35·0	45·6	45·3
Female	65·0	54·4	54·7
2. AGE			
Under 40	18·0	24·2	26·8
40–70	43·6	63·7	54·1
Over 70	38·4	12·1	19·1
3. CONDITION OF TREATMENT*			
Voluntary	71·8	20·2	76·7
Temporary	·6	—	—
Certified	27·6	79·8	23·3
4. TIME-LAPSE SINCE FIRST ADMISSION TO ANY MENTAL HOSPITAL (to date)			
Under 6 months	19·1	5·5	35·0
6 months—2 years	17·5	6·3	18·6
2–5 years	14·2	7·7	12·2
5–20 years	25·6	43·8	24·7
Over 20 years	23·6	36·7	9·5
5. LONG-STAY AND SHORT-STAY PATIENTS			
Long-stay	53·2	82·1	66·7
Short-stay	46·8	17·9	33·3
6. OCCUPATIONAL CLASS (men only)†			
Class I (professional, managerial)	60·5	3·2	16·6
Class II (inspecting, supervisory)	38·5	10·0	54·4
Class III (manual, routine non-manual)	1·0	86·8	29·0

* The census was taken before the introduction of informal status under the Mental Health Act 1959. There were at the time no de-designated beds in any of the three hospitals.

† This section is based on the Hall-Jones classification. See Methodology, Appendix I.

	Percentage of standing population		
	Crown Lodge	Northtown	Moordale
7. FINANCIAL STATUS			
Private	81·9	—	6·2
Amenity	—	—	49·7
Ministry of Pensions	5·1	—	—
Health Service	13·0	100·0	44·1

would thus reveal differences in basic needs and in organizational aims. A patient-census was carried out early in 1959, and provided the information in Table 5.

These figures indicate that there are very marked differences in the types of patients who go to the three hospitals. It was previously noted that there was a preponderance of female patients at Crown Lodge, and Section (1) of the Table confirms this—the proportion is roughly two women to one man, while at Northtown and Moordale, where the figures are very similar, it is six women to five men.

'*Classification by age*' (2) shows that Crown Lodge has many more elderly patients than the other two hospitals. Northtown surprisingly has the lowest proportion of over-seventies. This may be due to a lower expectation of life among Class III patients (see below).

'*Condition of treatment*' (3) shows that Crown Lodge and Moordale both have a high proportion of voluntary patients. Northtown by contrast has nearly 80 per cent still detained under certification. This may reflect the hospital's policy; or the pessimistic attitude of local mental welfare officers at the time of admission; or patients' own reactions to the prospect of entering a hospital of this type; or the types of patients admitted. Many come from the dock areas of a large port, and some are immigrants.

'*Time-lapse since first admission*' (4) relates to the earliest date found on patients' records, and does not necessarily imply that the patient has been in hospital continuously since that date, though this was so in the majority of cases, particularly those of long standing. In a few cases, patients may have previously been in other mental hospitals without our knowledge; but when previous admission was known to the hospital authorities, details were given in the case-file, and taken into account in our classification. The table indicates broadly the kind of cases treated in each hospital—whether these are of recent onset or of long duration. Crown Lodge has nearly 50 per cent, and Northtown 80 per cent, of patients first admitted more than five years ago. Moordale has only just over 30 per cent in this category, and by contrast, a very high proportion of cases of recent onset.

'Long-stay and short-stay patients' (5). It is very difficult to define theoretically the difference between these two categories. It is often assumed that a long-stay patient is one who has been in hospital continuously for more than two years; or that a long-stay patient is one for whom the prognosis is poor—a person who will probably have to stay in hospital for the rest of his or her life. Neither of these definitions can be related clearly to a standing population. Among those patients who have not yet been in hospital for eighteen months, there are almost certainly some whose eventual stay will be longer than that period, and we cannot with accuracy forecast which patients these are, or how many of them there will be. Prognosis again presents difficulties, for methods of treatment alter, and whether a patient is discharged often depends not on his clinical condition, but on the nature of his home circumstances.

In practice, however, psychiatrists distinguish between long-stay and short-stay patients every day. As we have seen, long-stay wards and short-stay wards are organized very differently, according to the needs of the patients and the degree of observation required. Section (5) is therefore based on the classification of the psychiatrists at the hospitals: long-stay patients are those on long-stay wards, and short-stay patients are those on short-stay wards. Medical superintendents were asked which wards were 'long-stay' in character, and which wards were 'short-stay', and the numbers of beds in each category were added for the hospital as a whole. These figures, which show a heavy concentration of long-stay beds at Northtown, form the basis of calculations in Chapter IX.

Occupational class (6) is not necessarily a measure of social class where mental patients are concerned. Schizophrenic patients, for example, are often found following Class III occupations although they have Class I family backgrounds, and this may account in part for the belief that schizophrenia has a higher incidence among the lower social groups.[1] Nor is it a reliable guide to income, since it is quite possible for a skilled manual worker to earn more than a clergyman or a young doctor or barrister. It is, however, a measure of the degree of social responsibility involved in previous work. Class I occupations are those which involve organizing one's own time, and that of employees, voluntary workers or other people. Class II occupations, such as those of foremen or inspectors, involve a lesser degree of responsibility.

Class III occupations involve working under supervision, without responsibility for the work of others.

It was not useful to classify women patients according to occupational class, since records in all three hospitals listed the occupation of a married woman as 'housewife' unless she had paid employment of her own, and no indication of the husband's occupation was given. Classification of the male patients (6) shows differences which are probably paralleled on the female side. At Crown Lodge, well over half the men were in Class I occupations, and Class III accounted for a mere one per cent. At Northtown, the overwhelming proportion were Class III, and Class I accounted only for a very small proportion. At Moordale, as one might expect from the three-fold system of admission, the population was more evenly distributed between the three groups.

'*Financial status*' (7) shows a position which has already been noted in dealing with each hospital in turn: at Crown Lodge, there is a high proportion of private patients. Health Service patients occupied 13 per cent of beds at the time when the census was taken; but, as explained in Chapter II, this proportion varies, since it is calculated in annual bed-days. At Moordale, the position is as noted in Table 3. At Northtown, all beds are for Health Service patients, and there is no provision for pay-beds.

It would be valuable to know whether the patients in the three hospitals differed in diagnostic categories; but no reliable information could be gained on this point. Pasamanick, Dinitz

[1] See Hollingshead and Redlich, 'Social Class and Mental Illness', 1958, and S. L. Morrison, *J. Ment. Sci.*, October 1959. Where this situation was encountered, patients were classified according to father's occupation, not according to their own at the time of admission to hospital, since the latter was probably a result of the onset of schizophrenia.

and Lefton,[1] in a recent American study, have shown that a group of psychiatrists with a common treatment orientation, working together in one hospital, can make diagnoses on the same group of patients which commonly differ by 20 per cent of the group, and may differ by as much as 50 per cent. We were therefore forced to the conclusion that, whatever system of classification was used, the compilation of figures from diagnoses by different doctors of different orientation, when referring to different groups of patients in different hospitals, would have been quite meaningless. The only solution would have been to ask one psychiatrist to re-diagnose all the cases[2]—an impossible task in view of the distances between the hospitals, and the numbers of patients involved.

In studying case-records, we came to the conclusion that the medical staff in the three hospitals did not diagnose in the same terms. At Northtown, there is a tendency to use a short label—'schizophrenia', 'manic-depression'. At Crown Lodge, diagnoses often take account both of the illness and the patient's basic personality, e.g. 'involutional depression in an immature personality'. At Moordale, multidimensional diagnoses covering several lines of the case-record are used by some doctors, and there is often an academic hesitation in giving a firm diagnosis at all. It was therefore very difficult to find any system of classification which could be used for all three hospitals. We have not attempted this with the patient-census, where large numbers of patients were involved; though, by reading full case-records and consulting medical staff in individual cases, we have attempted a simple form of classification for the much smaller numbers involved in the follow-up study (see p. 149).[3]

As far as the standing populations of the hospital are concerned, we have to be content with evidence drawn from the factors which were susceptible to measurement or observation.

[1] B. Pasamanick, S. Dinitz and M. Lefton, 'Psychiatric Orientation and its Relation to Diagnosis and Treatment in a Mental Hospital', *Am. J. Psych.*, 116/2, August 1959.

[2] The method suggested by Professor D. D. Reid (*Epidemiological Methods in the Study of Mental Disorders*, World Health Organization, 1960, p. 69).

[3] This is an even simpler classification than that recommended by Lemkau (*Am. J. Psych.*, 81/3, 1955). Section V of the International Classification of Diseases (W.H.O. 1948) lists 26 separate categories of mental illness. This was too detailed for a small-scale survey.

Crown Lodge has the greatest proportion of elderly patients, and therefore probably of patients suffering from senile psychoses. Northtown has the greatest proportion of long-stay patients—eighty per cent having entered mental hospital for the first time more than five years ago. It is reasonable to assume that this means the presence of many chronic patients, probably with a high incidence of schizophrenia. Moordale has many patients of recent admission, and in view of the age-structure at this hospital, we might expect that many of these patients would be suffering from early or mild degrees of mental disorder. With the exception of these general observations, we cannot make any comment on diagnostic categories.

The general picture given by the patient-census is as follows: Crown Lodge has a patient-population which is mainly elderly, mainly female, and predominantly from the upper occupational classes. Most patients entered hospital of their own accord, and could leave if they wished. The work thus falls into two categories: care for the very old or very demented; and group therapy on 'therapeutic community' lines for co-operative patients, who are used to making decisions and sitting on committees in the course of their normal occupational pursuits.

Northtown's population is very different: it is predominantly a community of long-stay, certified, working-class patients. They probably have less faith in authority and its workings than the patients at Crown Lodge—perhaps with justification, for it is a different type of authority and they stand in a different relation to it. Even in a time of universal primary education, they probably verbalize less easily, and are unused to taking major decisions for themselves, or to discussing matters of policy. They require a planned programme of activity if they are not to vegetate, and they would not take easily to the conditions of the 'therapeutic community' as practised at Crown Lodge.

At Moordale, the population is evenly balanced between age and occupation groups in comparison with the other two hospitals. There is a high proportion of voluntary patients, and a very high proportion of recent admissions. For these reasons, it is an excellent hospital for teaching purposes, and for the use of differing methods of psychiatric treatment in a single setting.

It is evident that the form of organization employed in each hospital is clearly related to the nature of the patient-population.

The needs of the patient-population to some extent dictate the shape of the hospital's work.

(*b*) *The aims of treatment.* These are capable of sub-division in two ways. First, the treatment of short-stay patients generally differs from that of long-stay patients. In one case, patients are being prepared for a return to ordinary life, with the responsibilities of family ties and employment. They may be acutely ill while they are in hospital; and we shall show later that short-stay patients make much greater demands on the hospital's resources in medical time, nursing time and drugs and dressings than long-stay patients do. Long-stay patients, whether they are treated actively or merely given custodial care, are suffering from chronic illness. The whole tempo of life on their wards is different from that on the short-stay wards. Return to life in the community is a fairly remote possibility for most of them, and in any case will depend more on adjustments in the conditions of community life than on improvements in their mental condition. Thus any mental hospital is providing two types of patient-care, very different in quality; and the proportion of long-stay patients to short-stay patients affects the demand for resources.

Second, the aim with regard to short-stay patients may vary according to the hospital's relationship with out-patient clinics, day hospitals and local authority Mental Health Services in the area. Crown Lodge, as an independent hospital, has few links with the community services. There is no social worker; referrals are not made to local authority Mental Health Departments; the hospital uses its own out-patient clinic in the grounds, but has no machinery for passing on to other agencies, apart from the general practitioner, patients who are unable to come back for further treatment. It follows that the aim at Crown Lodge must be to secure complete, or nearly complete, recovery before the patient is discharged.

Northtown and Moordale are in the Health Service, and situated in areas where community services have improved considerably since 1948. Both have social workers; both regularly make referrals on discharge, not only to the general practitioner, but also to the local authority; both have on their staff psychiatrists who conduct out-patient clinics, so that patients can be seen by a hospital psychiatrist at a clinic near their own homes. Provided that the patient's home circumstances are suitable, he may be discharged early in the convalescent stage, when he is still in need of care and treatment, but no longer in need of full in-patient services.

(*c*) *Other aims of mental hospital organization.* Any 'social organization', to use Talcott Parsons' term for an artificially-created human group, must devote a certain proportion of its resources to its own maintenance and perpetuation. Such activities as cleaning, re-decorating and the replacement of obsolescent equipment are a legitimate part of the hospital's work, even though they may benefit future patients rather than those who are in the hospital at the time.

Teaching functions are a valuable part of the work of a mental hospital. Conferences, staff meetings, study leave, study groups, and leave for senior staff to read papers to learned societies are all time-consuming activities which reduce the amount of time available for treating patients here and now. They may benefit patients in that hospital in the future, by improving staff skills and techniques; but they may not benefit patients in that hospital at all, for the hospital which has good training facilities attracts ambitious staff, and thus has a high staff turnover.

This can be illustrated from the three hospitals. At Northtown, which has minimal teaching functions, and where further study is not actively encouraged, the turnover in medical staff in the period June 1958–June 1959 was nil. At Crown Lodge, where teaching and therapy are closely interwoven, it was 2/6. At Moordale, where there is a direct link with university teaching, it was 3/6. One doctor at Crown Lodge and two at Moordale moved on promotion.

Such teaching activities are rightly regarded as part of the hospital's work, for they contribute to the raising of standards in the Mental Health Services as a whole; but they involve the immediate diversion of some of the hospital's resources away from the primary function of treating patients, and may, through increasing staff turnover, reduce continuity in care.

Hospital Status

Further differences between the hospitals arise from the separate and independent status of Crown Lodge. This is a limiting factor in that it prevents the hospital from making full use of the community services; but there are also inherent advantages. The medical staff at Crown Lodge can work full-time with their own patients. Senior medical staff do not have extra-mural responsibilities, and in-patients therefore receive more care from senior psychiatrists than is possible in Health Service hospitals.

Another advantage lies in ease of decision-making. When the medical superintendent and the Board of Management decided to build an occupational therapy centre, it was planned, built, opened and in operation within six months of the original decision. This is in marked contrast to the fate of a similar proposal at Moordale,[1] where the gap between the idea and execution will probably be twenty-one years. Even making allowances for the war years and post-war shortages, this is a very long time.

Crown Lodge is not subject to public accountability, and consequently enjoys greater freedom in the disposition of its resources. The use of an independent catering organization, the renting of the farm, and the sporadic employment of cleaning and decorating staff would be less easy under Health Service conditions, and there is no parallel at either Moordale or Northtown, which are bound to the mechanisms of Ministry consent and annual appropriations.

Crown Lodge is extremely sensitive to changing conditions. Financial insecurity is a powerful spur to flexibility. The development of the sheltered workshop, the plans for a day hospital, and other schemes for future development are closely related to the hospital's continuing need to adapt. Moordale has developed new research interests through contact with the university, on different lines. Northtown has little incentive to develop new interests with its present population-structure.

Hospital Size

For at least a hundred years, the small mental hospital of 400–800 beds has been upheld as the ideal. Lord Shaftesbury, as Chairman of the Lunacy Commissioners, was of this opinion in 1859.[2] The Expert Committee of the World Health Organization, in 1953, put the optimum at between 250 and 400

[1] See p. 99.

[2] *Report of Select Committee on Lunacy*, 1859.

beds.[1] The reason why so many hospitals of 1,000 or 2,000 or 3,000 beds developed between the two dates has little to do with ideals or optimum standards. This happened because mental hospital finance was until 1948 largely a local authority concern; and it was always cheaper to add wards to an existing hospital than to build a small new one.

No voices are raised in defence of the large hospital. For this reason, it is perhaps necessary to repeat that Northtown's large size does have certain advantages, notably in bulk buying and in the employment of specialist staff. The disadvantages of rigidity in administration, and the impossibility of preserving individuality for large masses of patients are, however, overwhelming.

The sociologist Charles S. Cooley first pointed out in 1909[2] that there is a fundamental difference in operation between the primary social group, consisting of not more than a few hundred people, and the secondary social group, consisting of several thousand. In a primary social group, individuality is preserved, because members of the group can meet in face-to-face relationships. In a secondary social group, individuality is lost, because the numbers are too great for all members of the community to meet in this way.

Secondary social groups are subject to fragmentation. The whole group is too big, and has too little meaning, to command the full loyalty of the members; and thus lesser loyalties take their place. In a mental hospital, these usually follow occupational lines, and the largest groups (doctors and nurses) exert the greatest pressure.

In these circumstances, role becomes more important than personality. Instead of Nurse Smith looking after Mrs. Brown, Mrs. Jones and Mrs. Robinson, ten nameless nurses superintend a hundred nameless patients. Quantity, as always, alters quality; and the quality of mental hospital care cannot be as good in these circumstances as in the intimate and personal setting of a small hospital. We cannot preserve the patient's sense of his own identity, encourage his self-respect, and help him to make genuine personal relationships with others if he is treated as one of a crowd.

[1] *Third Report of Expert Committee on Mental Health*, 953, p. 29.

[2] C. S. Cooley, *Social Organization*, p. 23 et seq.

This factor was observed in mental hospital life before the development of sociology as an academic discipline. Dr. Mortimer Grenville, Chairman of the *Lancet* Commission on Asylums wrote in 1877: 'It is only in small asylums that this potent remedy, the sane will working quietly on the insane, can be applied.'

The inherent handicaps of the large mental hospital have been observed at Northtown; and the inherent advantages of the small one emerge clearly from the studies at Crown Lodge and Moordale. This is a major factor of difference between the hospitals.

History and Tradition

'The most important single factor in the efficacy of treatment in a mental hospital,' write the World Health Organization's Expert Committee,[1] 'appears . . . to be an intangible element which can only be described as its atmosphere.' 'Atmosphere', they continue, is created by the nature of the relationships existing between staff and staff, staff and patients, and ultimately patients and patients.

This is certainly true; but the best staff cannot create the right relationships in the wrong setting. Mental hospitals, like individuals, cannot altogether make a fresh start at any point in time. They carry with them in the present all the associations of past successes and failures.

Hospitals, like individuals, do not even start life with a *tabula rasa*. The purpose for which the hospital was built, and the buildings which express that purpose, have an enduring influence. They create stereotypes, perhaps not consciously formulated, in the minds of both staff and patients. The nurse whose impression is 'This place is like an hotel' will behave towards her patients very differently from the nurse whose impression is 'This place is like a prison'. Patients are similarly affected by the impression which the hospital makes on them, and will behave like patrons or like prisoners accordingly.[2]

[1] *Op. cit.*, p. 17.

[2] For a consideration of the effect of architecture in creating mental hospital stereotypes, see P. Sivadon, 'Mental Health Problems in Hospitals', *International Social Science Journal*, U.N.E.S.C.O., Vol. XI, No. I, 1959, and H. Osmund, *Function as a Basis for Ward Design* (unpublished, privately circulated, 1956).

Because of the importance of this factor of 'atmosphere', we feel that it may be worth recording our own impressions of the three hospitals in the survey. These are highly subjective; but we believe that this is the kind of judgement which staff and patients often make, and which conditions their behaviour towards one another.

Crown Lodge is like an hotel. The buildings are mellow and pleasant, the service is first class, and staff, particularly nursing staff, are often deferential to patients, many of whom are wealthier, and come from higher social strata than they themselves do. Patients often make their own amusement as they would in a spa or hydro—reading, playing bridge, walking in the grounds or the surrounding country, or talking in small groups over a cup of coffee.

Northtown creates two quite distinct impressions. The walls, the gates, the corridors, the locked doors, and the depressed-looking long-stay patients who drift aimlessly about corridors or grounds, make one think of a Victorian Poor Law Institution. The short-stay wards, particularly the new ones, are more like good, well-kept youth hostels. The staff are on the whole kind to the patients, but tend to act in a superior, supervisory role. Many of the long-stay patients are thoroughly institutionalized, assimilated to the routine. Short-stay patients can fill in the time pleasantly if they like mass life, and are not too resentful of authority.

Moordale is like a village. It is a close-knit little community, rather given to gossip and rumours, where everybody takes an intense interest in the doings of everybody else. Staff and patients tend to meet as equals, though the medical superintendent is much respected as the head of the community. Newcomers are greeted with great interest and friendliness, and quickly incorporated into 'village' activities.

The stereotype of the general hospital would not readily occur to an observer in any of the three hospitals, except on the sick wards. Here, in all three, there is a high standard of professional care, and the atmosphere is very much that of a good general hospital ward; but with this exception, the three hospitals are very different in 'atmosphere'.

Psychiatric Orientation

Unlike general hospitals, where procedure in most specialisms is highly standardized, mental hospitals differ tremendously in orientation. It is possible to find hospitals where psychotherapy is frowned upon as 'time-wasting', and all treatment is by organic methods. At others, physical treatment is used hardly at all, and has been succeeded by 'education in group living' which lays great stress on behaviour patterns and individual and group reactions.

None of the three hospitals goes quite to the extremes which can be found elsewhere in England; but treatment at Northtown is almost entirely on organic lines—partly because there is no time for psychotherapy, and partly because the hospital can support excellent laboratory and pharmaceutical services on the spot. At Crown Lodge, much emphasis is laid on group therapy on therapeutic community lines though organic methods of treatment are used in conjunction with individual and group therapy in most cases; and at Moordale, a variety of emphases are found, according to the individual doctor's training and experience. It is probable that doctors at Moordale could talk psychiatry with doctors at either Crown Lodge or Northtown without great difficulty; but doctors at Crown Lodge and Northtown might find it difficult to talk to each other. It is not merely that they refer to different kinds of experience. Quite often, they do not even use the same kind of technical vocabulary.

Administrative Patterns

Crown Lodge and Northtown, for all their differences in approach, have one situation at least in common: both are self-contained units, functioning under a basically centralized form of administration. Moordale is not self-contained, being now very closely associated with other hospitals in the group, and authority in the day-to-day running of the hospital is diffused.

The Health Service—and the Future

The inception of the Health Service meant very different things to the three hospitals. To Crown Lodge, Health Service administration was a threat to be avoided. To Northtown, it was the beginning of a great opportunity. To Moordale, it was something very like occupation by a foreign power. In all three hospitals, the implications of change are still being worked out.

At Crown Lodge, total bed-occupation has begun to drop since 1957, though admission rates have risen. This is part of a general trend in mental hospitals, for methods of treatment, both organic and psychodynamic, have improved greatly, and patients generally stay in hospital for much shorter periods than they did in pre-war days. To many Health Service hospitals, such a small but progressive decrease in the size of the standing population means a relief from the problems of waiting lists and serious overcrowding. To a small independent hospital, the situation is a paradoxical one: more efficient treatment means speedier discharge for short-stay patients, a smaller standing population, and hence a smaller income. This could mean a threat to the survival of Crown Lodge, for, as a charitable institution, the hospital does not create substantial financial reserves.

Unless the hospital constantly adapts to fresh demands, it could face financial difficulties in the future. It is no longer as easy as it once was to raise public subscriptions, and Crown Lodge could ironically become a self-liquidating institution.

Northtown has seen many improvements since the Appointed Day. Again, the present position is a transitional one, for there is still much which could be done; but the future of old 'county asylums' such as Northtown is doubtful. It may be that, with the increase of community work, and the development of small psychiatric centres at general hospitals, hospitals of this type will gradually be allowed to fall into disuse. In the meantime, the staff continue to combat the effects of poor and depressing buildings, public prejudice, and a huge institutionalized population. The medical superintendent points out that both Crown Lodge and Moordale can select their patients to some extent—fee-paying in itself involves some degree of self-selection among patients. He has no choice: among his patients can be found not only the problems of mental illness, but the problems of squalor and ignorance and acute poverty. The needs are great; the resources, even now, quite inadequate.

Moordale, despite its administrative problems, is in a favourable position compared to the other two hospitals; for it has public prestige combined with material security. It is firmly based on the local community, closely associated with a centre of teaching and research. The transitional period has not been an easy one, but it is drawing to a close. There seems no reason why the hospital should not continue on present lines, and there is no threat of closure either on the grounds of financial instability or of general unsuitability for modern psychiatric work.

The three hospitals are thus quite different from each other in character. That they show marked differentiation on a number of criteria is not merely fortuitous. To use medical terminology, we are confronted with three syndromes, rather than three sets of unrelated symptoms.

They differ from each other both in needs and in resources, and there is no valid base-line for total comparison. It might therefore be contended that it is quite impossible to compare them in any way; but in practice, comparisons are frequently made between mental hospitals, and must continue to be made, for service planning is impossible unless some standards of comparison can be found. If sound criteria for comparison cannot be evolved, comparisons will be made on unsound ones.

In the next three chapters, we consider a number of commonly employed 'measures of efficiency' in relation to the three hospitals, and make our own proposals for a limited measure which avoids most of the pitfalls created by the wide differences which have been described.

VI

SIMPLE MEASURES OF EFFICIENCY—I

SIMPLE measures of efficiency usually attempt to assess the totality of work done by the results of one part of that work. The part chosen for such a measure is generally one which is readily accessible, and which can be expressed in quantitative terms. In mental hospitals, the measures which have commonly been taken as an index of efficiency are:

1. The condition of patients on discharge—i.e. the proportion of 'cures' or recoveries.
2. The admission rate.
3. The discharge rate.
4. Staff ratios.
5. Medical clinical time.
6. The average length of stay for discharged patients.
7. The relapse rate.
8. Average cost.

Each of these measures has its own limitations, and these will be discussed, figures from Crown Lodge, Northtown, and Moordale being used in illustration.

1. *Condition on discharge*

As institutions for the treatment of mental illness developed in the early nineteenth century, medical superintendents made a practice of ending their annual reports with statistics of patients 'cured'. This seemed an obvious and satisfactory way of expressing a hospital's efficiency, and a justification for its work.

Figures published at this time were very unreliable. At Hanwell Asylum, it was claimed in the eighteen-thirties that 90 per cent of patients admitted were discharged 'cured'. This claim drew forth a series of trenchant comments from Dr. Caleb Crowther, medical superintendent of the West Riding Asylum, who exposed some 'Fallacies and Tricks employed at some Lunatic Asylums to make the apparent Number of Cures greater than the Real Number'.[1] Patients discharged 'care of friends' were listed as 'cured', whatever their real condition on discharge. Patients readmitted after 'cure' were listed as fresh cases. The labouring poor of the county of Middlesex were much given to gin-drinking, and Hanwell admitted many drunken patients, discharging them as soon as they were sober—'These are fine cases for swelling statistical reports and deceiving the public', wrote Crowther.

> In no hospital in Europe, even when appropriated solely to recent cases, have ninety out of one hundred patients ever been cured, and as long as the present state of society and manners lasts, we may safely predict never will.

He pointed out that few hospitals could take only recent or early cases. Many patients were incurable on admission, and many so physically frail that a high mortality rate was inevitable. The proportion of such cases would vary from hospital to hospital, according to the locality, and would affect the proportion of patients who could be discharged 'cured'.

Psychiatrists no longer speak of 'cures', for they recognize that a state of perfect mental health is an abstraction, and tend to prefer the term 'recovered'. Patients are classified on discharge as 'recovered', 'relieved' and 'not improved', and comparative statistics could be compiled from these classifications; but some of Caleb Crowther's arguments against the use of this measure still hold good, and there are other reasons also why it may be inappropriate.

Whether a patient has 'recovered'—and from what—is a relative judgement, and at least in part a matter of personal

[1] C. Crowther, *Observations on the Management of Madhouses, illustrated by Occurrences in the West Riding and Middlesex Asylums*, Simpkin Marshall, London, 1838.

opinion. There is no clear-cut test which can be employed, and opinions will often differ from psychiatrist to psychiatrist.

A decision as to classification on discharge may be influenced by extraneous factors, such as the patient's length of stay in hospital. If he discharges himself after two days, he is almost certainly 'not improved' in relation to his condition at the time of admission, because the hospital has had no time in which to improve that condition. If he has been in hospital for three or four months, some psychiatrists, acting on the assumption that psychiatric treatment is beneficial to psychiatric patients, may be tempted to describe him as 'relieved' or 'recovered'.

The moment of discharge is not a suitable one for making a judgement on the patient's condition; for he is about to leave a known environment, in which his reactions have been observed, for the unknown stresses of life in the community. Whether he does in fact recover may depend more on what the community at large does to him than on what the hospital has done for him. In order to illustrate this point, we compared the condition on discharge of a sample[1] of patients from the three hospitals with their actual condition two years later:

TABLE 6

Condition of Random Sample of Patients on Discharge measured against subsequent Readmission to Mental Hospital (percentage)

	Crown Lodge	Northtown	Moordale
'Recovered' on discharge	45·0	39·6	27·8
subsequently readmitted	11·0	5·9	6·8
'Relieved' on discharge	48·0	44·5	66·2
subsequently readmitted	19·0	18·7	20·3
'Not improved' on discharge	7·0	15·9	6·0
subsequently readmitted	2·0	7·0	1·5

In each case, a substantial proportion of patients discharged 'recovered' entered a mental hospital again within two years of discharge, while the majority of those 'not improved' on

[1] This will be referred to hereafter as 'the random sample'. It consisted of 100 patients from Crown Lodge, 101 from Northtown and 132 from Moordale discharged September 1956–March 1957. These were randomly selected, except that multiple admissions and cases of known organic origin were discarded. See pp. 147 and 195.

discharge did not. The hospitals' estimate of condition on discharge is thus shown to bear no direct relation to patients' subsequent progress.

We conclude, therefore, that statistics compiled on this basis are valueless for the purpose of assessing the work of mental hospitals.

2. *The admission rate*

In the nineteen-thirties, when the Mental Treatment Act was coming into effect, and voluntary patients began to be admitted to mental hospitals, the admission rate was often treated as being of great significance. A mental hospital with a high admission rate was, to borrow a phrase from an allied field, a 'flowing stream' rather than a 'stagnant pool'.[1] It was felt that such a hospital was overcoming the stigma which still prevented so many people from seeking mental treatment, and thus serving the community better than a hospital with a static population and a low admission rate.

This attitude rested on the assumption—justified at the time—that there were many people who needed mental treatment and did not come forward to receive it. Other medical and social services have passed through a similar period. In the early part of the twentieth century, for example, a similar stress was placed on ascertainment in the tuberculosis, blind welfare, and mental deficiency services. There is a stage at which a service has been provided, and the main task is to make contact with those who need to make use of it; but this stage soon passes, to be replaced by an emphasis on treatment and discharge.

This has now happened as far as mental hospitals are concerned. With the increase in community care, and the greater willingness of the general public to seek treatment when necessary, admission figures have become largely irrelevant to the work which hospitals do. In all mental hospitals, admission rates have increased; but this is not only because empty beds are being filled, or new ones provided. It is because treatment has improved, discharge rates have increased, and so beds become vacant more quickly. This is a change of tempo, not a change in scope. How fast the tempo has increased depends on

[1] Used by the Report of the Wood Committee, 1929, in reference to mental deficiency hospitals.

TABLE 7

Admission Rates, 1945–57

	Admissions	Resident Population	Percentage Admissions over Resident Population
1. CROWN LODGE			
1945	404	368	109·8
1946	397	345	115·1
1947	370	328	112·8
1948	429	323	132·8
1949	395	327	120·8
1950	354	335	105·7
1951	352	316	111·4
1952	439	328	133·8
1953	477	357	133·6
1954	563	383	147·0
1955	648	375	172·8
1956	637	387	164·6
1957	637	365	174·5
2. NORTHTOWN			
1945	538	2935	18·3
1946	563	2957	19·0
1947	501	2920	17·1
1948	705	2935	24·0
1949	902	2892	31·1
1950	858	2852	30·0
1951	1068	2799	38·2
1952	1045	2799	37·3
1953	1078	2756	39·1
1954	1082	2758	39·2
1955	1126	2766	40·7
1956	1208	2789	43·3
1957	1217	2708	44·9
3. MOORDALE			
1945	276	264	104·5
1946	316	273	115·7
1947	307	265	115·9
1948	354	264	134·1
1949	426	247	172·4
1950	317	250	126·8
1951	350	260	134·6
1952	392	279	140·5
1953	396	292	135·6
1954	420	309	135·9
1955	437	308	141·9
1956	429	332	129·2
1957	594	372	159·7

the number of beds blocked by long-stay patients; for one patient who stays in hospital for 20 years occupies a bed which could serve 80 patients staying for three months each.

It will be noted that all three hospitals show a considerable increase in admissions between 1945 and 1957. The *proportionate* increase is greater at Northtown (from 18·3 to 44·9 per cent) than at Crown Lodge (109·8 to 174·5 per cent) or Moordale (104·5 to 159·7 per cent), though the numbers of patients involved are much smaller. In all three hospitals, a sharp upward trend started in 1948, reflecting the increasing turnover since that time.

At Northtown, the standing population has dropped during this period by over 200. At Crown Lodge, it is almost the same as it was in 1945, though it shows signs of decreasing now. At Moordale, it has increased rapidly in the last few years—not because the hospital is failing to cure its patients, but because it is Regional Board policy to increase its size. The shortage of space at Moordale has been commented on in Chapter III.

Admission figures are of interest in considering general patterns of hospital development, and often illustrate policy changes. Taken by themselves, they can be misleading, and cannot be considered as an adequate index of efficiency.

3. *The discharge rate*

We have now passed beyond the 'period of ascertainment', and today, medical superintendents and lay administrators are more likely to boast of high discharge rates than of high admission rates. The Royal Commission on Mental Illness and Mental Deficiency, 1954–7, and the Mental Health Act, 1959, both emphasize the importance of getting mental hospital patients out into the community. The hospital which can discharge the most patients in the shortest time is often spoken of as the most efficient—without reference to the number of patients fit to be discharged, or the conditions to which they return. Such a policy has its dangers. Patients who figure in the discharge lists may well figure more than once in subsequent admission lists.[1] To

[1] Miss Eileen Brooke (*J. Ment. Sci.*, 105/411, October 1959) has criticized the common use of admission and discharge statistics on the grounds that such statistics '. . . have not told us who is ill, but how many times the swing door . . . has opened for someone to pass through'.

TABLE 8

Discharge Rates, 1945–57

	Discharges	Resident Population	Discharges over Resident Population
1. CROWN LODGE			
1945	339	368	92·1
1946	374	345	108·4
1947	339	328	103·3
1948	389	323	120·4
1949	341	327	104·3
1950	306	335	91·3
1951	329	316	104·1
1952	374	328	114·0
1953	374	357	104·8
1954	460	383	120·1
1955	592	375	157·9
1956	596	387	154·0
1957	593	365	162·5
2. NORTHTOWN			
1945	370	2935	12·6
1946	334	2957	11·3
1947	404	2920	13·8
1948	646	2935	22·0
1949	742	2892	25·7
1950	785	2852	27·5
1951	894	2799	31·9
1952	898	2799	32·0
1953	1033	2756	37·5
1954	954	2758	34·6
1955	1018	2766	36·8
1956	1178	2789	42·2
1957	1190	2708	43·9
3. MOORDALE			
1945	240	265	90·9
1946	286	273	104·8
1947	282	265	106·4
1948	339	264	128·4
1949	400	247	161·9
1950	321	250	128·4
1951	287	260	110·4
1952	347	279	124·4
1953	368	292	126·0
1954	376	309	121·7
1955	402	308	130·5
1956	407	332	122·6
1957	528	372	141·9

get a patient out of hospital does not necessarily mean that he will stay out, or that he will be better cared for than if he had remained in.

The general pattern of discharge statistics shows a clear similarity to that of admissions. Thus Crown Lodge had a year of unusually high admissions in 1948, and Moordale in 1949. These are also respectively years of unusually high discharges. Crown Lodge had an unusually low admission rate in 1949, and Moordale in 1956. These are also years of unusually low discharges. The two sets of figures are closely linked, for a mental hospital can only discharge those patients who have been admitted, and admit patients to replace those who have been discharged.

Again, the increase at Northtown, though much smaller in terms of the standing population, is proportionately greater. The figure rises from 12·6 in 1945 to 43·9 in 1957—more than a threefold increase. Crown Lodge's figure rises in the same period from 92·1 to 162·5, and Moordale's from 90·9 to 141·9 per cent.

The two small hospitals, as one might expect, show much more fluctuation than the large one.

Discharge rates, like admission rates, are very much at the mercy of extraneous influences. They tell us simply on how many occasions patients were discharged during a certain year. They show that there has been a greater volume of discharges at some hospitals than at others. The causes, circumstances or results of discharge remain unknown.

Another method of approach is to express discharges as a percentage of admissions (see Table 9, opposite).

This tends to show that, when its huge long-stay population is excluded from the calculation, Northtown's record is comparable with that of the other two hospitals.

On the whole, it is true to say that the patients who are admitted are also the patients who are discharged within the same year or the following one. The short-stay beds turn over rapidly, while the patient-population in long-stay beds is largely static.

There is, of course, a variable proportion of deaths at each hospital, and these also affect the beds vacated. If many old or physically sick patients are admitted, the difference between the

TABLE 9

Discharges Expressed as a Percentage of Admissions, 1945–57

	Crown Lodge	Northtown	Moordale
1945	83·9	68·8	87·0
1946	94·2	59·3	90·5
1947	91·6	80·6	91·9
1948	90·7	91·6	95·8
1949	86·3	82·3	93·9
1950	86·4	91·4	101·2
1951	93·5	83·7	82·0
1952	85·2	85·9	88·5
1953	78·4	95·8	92·9
1954	81·7	88·1	89·5
1955	91·4	90·4	92·0
1956	93·6	97·5	94·7
1957	93·1	97·8	88·9

discharge rate and the actual bed-vacation rate may be considerable.

It is a fair guess that any hospital discharging more than 95 per cent of the admission figure for a given year is tending to reduce its standing population; and that any hospital discharging less than 70 per cent is adding to it. These, however, are facts which can be ascertained much more easily by checking the standing population figures for successive years. All we have obtained from this additional calculation is a crude measure of bed turnover.

4. *Staff ratios*

Some clues to the work of a hospital can be obtained from a consideration of the numerical relationship of patients to staff. This is not always as simple to estimate as it appears superficially to be. Medical staff may have differing extra-mural commitments. Hospitals may employ differing proportions of junior and senior medical and nursing staff. Some hospitals employ more part-time nurses than others; and the equation of part-time nurses to full-time nurses (on the principle that two half-time nurses, for example, are equivalent to one full-time nurse) leaves out of consideration the extra time necessary for a hand-over between those going off duty and those taking over. When we come to consider social workers, occupational therapists, social therapists and other ancillary workers, the problem becomes more difficult, because these people do not have strictly defined roles. The social workers at Northtown and Moordale have a sphere of operation which does not seem to exist at Crown Lodge, because the doctors do the work, the necessity does not arise for it with well-to-do patients, or the work goes by default. The social therapists at Moordale do work which is shared between nursing staff and occupational therapists at the other two hospitals. Northtown has a full-time librarian. Library work at Crown Lodge is undertaken by a voluntary body (Red Cross and St. John) and at Moordale by the social therapists. There is thus a mixed group of duties in the social care of patients which is differently allocated in different hospitals, and which cannot be accurately measured by staff appointments.

TABLE 10

Staff Ratios in Relation to Resident Population (April 1959)

	Crown Lodge	Northtown	Moordale
Medical staff	1 : 37	1 : 130	1 : 56
Nursing staff	1 : 3	1 : 5·25	1 : 4
Social work staff	nil	1 : 917	1 : 400

Clearly, a greater amount of medical and nursing care can be provided at Crown Lodge for each patient than at the other two hospitals. In fact, the difference is greater than the figures suggest; for we know that Crown Lodge doctors have few extramural duties, and that the hospital employs few part-time nursing staff. Crown Lodge and Moordale, however, are both in a very favourable position in comparison with Northtown. Though Northtown's nursing ratio is better than that at many similar hospitals (where ratios of 1 : 8 or even 1 : 10 are not unknown), the medical ratio is low.

To say that Crown Lodge has one nurse to three patients, or Northtown one to 5·25, does not of course imply that this is the ward-strength at any given moment. When allowance is made for two day-shifts and a night-shift, and for days off, sick leave and holidays, the average number of patients dealt with by any one nurse is probably about three times as great. Since nursing staff are not evenly divided among the patients (they tend to be concentrated on sick-wards and those wards where intensive observation is necessary) some nurses will deal with many more.

Medical staff tend to be concentrated on the short-stay wards, as can be seen from the following section. At Northtown in particular, the long-stay patients receive little medical attention apart from routine physical care.

Staff ratios indicate gross differences in the staff available, and the amount of care available for patients. They do not show how hard or how long the staff work, or how their time is allocated. Nor do they give any indications of the calibre or grade of staff employed.

5. *Medical clinical time*

In recent years, some attempts have been made, though to our knowledge none have been published, to estimate the amount of time which psychiatrists in mental hospitals actually spend in the care of patients. Psychiatrists are understandably reticent on this score. As professional men, they feel that the allocation of their time is their own personal responsibility, and that their work cannot be adequately measured by the number of minutes spent on this duty and that.

Since much of their work involves confidential interviewing, it would not be possible to obtain a pattern of their activities from orthodox time and motion study methods. Estimates have consequently been hitherto based on psychiatrists' own estimates, often made considerably in arrears. A study undertaken by a committee of the Royal Medico-Psychological Association in 1959, for instance, had to base its findings on how much time psychiatrists estimated that they had spent on certain types of work in the previous year.

Medical staff at Crown Lodge, Northtown and Moordale were fortunately very co-operative, and we were able to obtain a day-by-day summary of each doctor's activities within the hospital over a 'test month'. The organization of this work is described in the appendix on methodology. Table 11 gives the average number of hours worked within the hospital by each doctor per week, and a breakdown under heads representing the main types of activity.

TABLE 11

Medical Staffs: Average Pattern of Employment (hours per week)

	Clinical care of Short-stay Patients	Clinical care of Long-stay Patients	General Admin.	Staff, etc. Meetings	Misc.	Total
CROWN LODGE						
Dr. A.	24	4	15	6	6	55
Dr. B.	34	9	0	2	1	46
Dr. C.	38	2	0	6	4	50
Dr. D.	46	0	0	3	0	49
Dr. E.	41	1	0	3	1	46
Dr. F.	3	33	0	0	0	36
Dr. G.	25	15	0	3	0	43
NORTHTOWN						
Dr. N.	0	0	37	3	0	40
Dr. O.	0	19	4	2	0	25
Dr. P.	3	8	5	2	6	24
Dr. Q.	28	0	8	3	1	40
Dr. R.	29	0	2	2	6	39
Dr. S.	24	1	4	1	0	30
Dr. T.	0	18	6	3	1	28
Dr. U.	0	39	3	0	0	42
Dr. V.	27	3	6	0	1	37
Dr. W.	5	16	7	1	2	31
Dr. X.	0	25	6	2	4	37
Dr. Y.	8	16	6	2	7	39
Dr. Z.	0	22	11	0	0	33
Dr. AA.	8	23	6	2	0	39
Dr. BB.	17	10	2	2	0	31
Dr. CC.	18	5	5	3	1	32
Dr. DD.	29	2	8	1	2	42
Dr. EE.	26	5	1	1	0	33
Dr. FF.	27	2	7	2	0	38
MOORDALE						
Dr. H.	11	10	5	2	0	28
Dr. I.	12	4	6	2	0	24
Dr. J.	21	6	1	0	5	33
Dr. K.	29	13	6	0	1	49
Dr. L.	16	7	6	5	7	41
Dr. M.	24	7	10	0	4	45

NOTES:

(1) Doctors in each hospital are arranged in descending order of salary.

(2) No account is taken in the table of time during which the doctors were 'on call', or of extra-mural work.

(3) 19 of the 22 doctors at Northtown completed time-sheets. Two were on sick leave throughout the 'test month', and one failed to make returns.

The average number of hours' work done per week within the hospital per doctor is thus 46·43 at Crown Lodge, 34·74 at Northtown, and 36·67 at Moordale. This may bear no relation to total hours worked at the two Health Service hospitals, since commitments outside the hospital vary from doctor to doctor, and also from time to time. Time 'on call' is greater at Crown Lodge and Moordale, which have small staffs, since one doctor must always be on duty, by day or night. At Northtown, one senior doctor and one junior doctor are generally 'on call' together, but since the total staff is larger, this duty is less frequent.

From Table 11, it is possible to calculate the average amount of clinical time spent with each patient per week. Again, these figures should be treated with caution, for the amounts will in fact vary greatly; but they provide a rough and ready measure of the amount of medical time spent in actual contact with patients (as distinct from time spent at staff meetings, in completing case-histories, dictating correspondence, and other duties).

TABLE 12

Analysis of Medical Clinical Time (in minutes)

	Crown Lodge	Northtown	Moordale
Average per short-stay patient per week	133·3	29·9	35·3
Average per long-stay patient per week	20·9	5·6	13·7

There is thus some justification for regarding medical care at Crown Lodge as 'intensive', and that at Northtown as 'minimal'.

In terms of the total medical clinical time available per patient, Crown Lodge is able to provide a much better service. Short-stay patients see their doctors for an average of more than two hours per week, compared to roughly half an hour at the other two hospitals, and long-stay patients also receive more care.

Crown Lodge has more medical time to allocate; but if we consider not the total amount of doctor-time available but the ways in which it is allocated between long-stay and short-stay patients, it will be seen that Crown Lodge and Northtown follow a similar policy, and Moordale a different one. At both Crown

Lodge and Northtown, there is a fairly heavy concentration on the needs of the short-stay patient. Moordale gives a higher proportion of doctor-time to the long-stay patient. This may reflect adversely on Moordale's discharge and length-of-stay figures, for these figures refer largely to short-stay patients. Mental hospitals are often in the position of having to rob Peter to pay Paul, any improvement in the care of one type of patient being made at the expense of the other.

VII

SIMPLE MEASURES OF EFFICIENCY—II

6. *Average length of stay*

If a patient recovers from his illness in four weeks at Hospital A., and we could show that the same patient would have taken four months to reach the same point in recovery at Hospital B., we would have a measure of efficiency which was at least satisfactory for patients suffering from that form and degree of illness; but these conditions are purely theoretical. In fact, hospitals are dealing with different patients at different stages in their illness, and treating them in different ways with differing results.

Personal factors greatly affect the length of stay of individual patients in an age of voluntary admissions. Possibly in Caleb Crowther's day, the length of stay had a real meaning; for patients then went into hospital under certification, and stayed until they were discharged. They left when the hospital was ready to discharge them, irrespective of the conditions to which they returned, for after-care was not yet even a theoretical concept. Today, the length of stay has no real relevance. Mrs. A. may enter hospital on Monday, decide that she does not want treatment, and go home on Thursday. On Saturday, she may be back again, in response to the urging of her husband and family doctor—to discharge herself again on the following Monday. Mr. B. may be well enough to leave hospital on a purely clinical criterion; but if he has no home to go to, or no employment to return to, he may stay in hospital until arrangements have been made for him. Miss C. may be an old lady who has been in hospital for many years. Suddenly, through a change in domestic circumstances, her relatives may be able to offer her a home, and ask for her discharge.

Crude length-of-stay figures refer to the time between admission and discharge of every patient discharged during a certain period irrespective of the reason of discharge, or the number of readmissions. Something can be done to refine them by limiting the calculation to 'first admissions'—that is, to patients who have only entered a mental hospital once. The following table gives the average length of stay for the random sample:

TABLE 13

Average Length of Stay (first admissions)

Crown Lodge	69·26 days	(S.D. = 56·26)
Northtown	114·64 days	(S.D. = 184·70)
Moordale	101·55 days	(S.D. = 156·73)

The standard deviations given above show that there is a very wide scatter, and that the average gives an impression of homogeneity which the figures do not in any way justify.

Patients who walk out of hospital after two or three days without receiving treatment shorten the average length of stay, thus giving the impression that the hospital is more 'efficient'. Conversely, if the hospital takes a great deal of trouble in resettling patients who have been in-patients for some years, the average length of stay is pushed up, and the hospital appears less 'efficient'.

Further refinement of the length-of-stay calculation, however, produces considerable problems. We cannot say with certainty that the patient who has been in hospital for a week or less has received no benefit from hospitalization; and a limitation on the length of stay (for instance, by considering only those patients discharged within two years of admission) would operate in favour of those hospitals which commonly keep patients over a long period.

In certain cases, such as those where a hospital has made a definite attempt to secure the discharge of long-stay patients to hostels or other accommodation, the exclusion of these patients from the length-of-stay calculation might be justified. In Crown

Lodge, Northtown and Moordale, this was not the case. Only three patients in the random sample (one at Moordale and two at Northtown) had been in hospital for more than two years, and the length of stay in all three instances was less than four years.

7. *The relapse rate*

Like the average length of stay, the relapse rate is concerned almost exclusively with short-stay patients. Long-stay patients form roughly half of the standing population at Crown Lodge and Moordale, and over four-fifths at Northtown. As far as these patients are concerned, apart from the measurement of the cost of their maintenance, 'efficiency' can be judged at present only in terms of their comfort and happiness—concepts which cannot be tested or measured statistically.

We are therefore concerned only with a proportion of the patients from the three hospitals, a proportion which varies from hospital to hospital. The question we are asking is not the sweeping 'Does this hospital cure its patients?' but the more limited 'What results do the facilities for short-stay patients at this hospital produce?' In effect, this means comparing the work of the short-stay wards at Crown Lodge and Moordale with that of the modernized units (Neurosis Unit, villas and female rehabilitation ward) at Northtown. This is a very different matter from comparing whole hospitals.

As we have shown earlier in this chapter, psychiatrists' own estimates of their patients' condition on discharge do not bear any relation to the actual relapse figures, as summarized two years later.

In that interim two-year period, many factors have had an influence on the patient's progress: an understanding and sympathetic family will cushion many of the strains of readjustment; a family where there is bitterness and stress in personal relationships may be the instrument of another breakdown. A simple manual form of employment may be far less taxing than a complex professional one, in which personal relationships with colleagues and mental lucidity are all-important. The stigma which still attaches to mental illness, with all that it implies in unhelpfulness, lack of sympathy, and positive, if unconscious, cruelty by friends and neighbours, may be a powerful factor in preventing recovery.

The patient's progress after discharge is also affected by the quality of the services which the community can offer in the immediate period of resettlement. General practitioners vary greatly in their knowledge of psychiatric disorder[1] and in the amount of time which they are able (or willing) to devote to patients discharged from mental hospital. Out-patient clinics, local authority mental health departments, and other social agencies are patchy both in distribution and quality. Though some County areas maintain a service of good quality, it is generally true that patients who live in a town are better cared for than those who live in remote rural areas.

A follow-up study was carried out by means of both a random sample and a matched group. These give different types of information. A random sample gives a typical picture of each hospital's work with short-stay patients; a matched sample gives a picture which is probably atypical for each hospital, but which enables comparisons to be made.

The random sample is the one referred to on page 125.

There is a wide distribution in age-groups (2) in all three cases. Patients discharged from Crown Lodge are on an average slightly older than those from the other two hospitals, and discharges from Northtown drop sharply after the age of 60. Moordale has the widest range in age. Although the majority of patients discharged are under 40, patients are discharged well into their fifties and sixties and some in their seventies.

As expected from the patient-census, the figures for occupation (3) show great differences between the hospitals. Over three-quarters of patients discharged from Northtown are manual or routine clerical workers, i.e. workers whose employment carries no real degree of responsibility. The surprisingly high figures for Classes II and III at Crown Lodge can be explained by the rapid turnover of National Health Service patients, who do not stay in the hospital for more than six months; but even so, to take the Class I figures, half the Crown Lodge patients go back to work of considerable responsibility,

[1] Dr. C. P. Blacker (*Neurosis and the Mental Health Services*, 1946) found that general practitioners' estimates of the proportion of illness among their patients due to psychiatric causes varied from 2 to 70 per cent.

TABLE 14

Composition of Random Sample

*Figures in percentages, to one decimal point**

	Crown Lodge	Northtown	Moordale
1. SEX			
Male	34·0	47·4	45·1
Female	66·0	52·6	54·9
2. AGE ON DISCHARGE			
under 20	5·0	4·0	2·2
20–29	14·0	28·7	18·8
30–39	23·0	23·7	20·3
40–49	25·0	19·8	24·8
50–59	21·0	17·8	22·6
60–69	10·0	5·0	11·3
70–79	2·0	1·0	0
80 and over	nil	nil	nil
3. OCCUPATIONAL CLASS (men only)			
Class I	50·0	6·2	25·0
Class II	38·2	14·6	31·7
Class III	11·8	79·2	43·3
4. FINANCIAL STATUS			
Private	66·0	0	9·0
Amenity	0	0	40·7
N.H.S.	34·0	100·0	50·3
5. HOSPITAL STATUS			
Voluntary	93·0	74·2	94·7
Temporary	1·0	1·0	·8
Certified	6·0	24·8	4·5
6. DIAGNOSIS			
Schizophrenia	30·0	25·7	15·8
Affective disorder	47·0	58·4	49·6
Mixed atypical	23·0	15·9	34·6
7. LENGTH OF STAY			
Under 7 days	2·0	3·0	3·0
8–31 days	19·0	19·8	25·6
32 days—6 months	77·0	63·3	60·0
6 months—2 years	2·0	11·9	10·6
Over 2 years	0	2·0	·8
8. CONDITION OF DISCHARGE (hospital's prognosis)			
Recovered	44·0	39·6	27·8
Relieved	48·0	44·5	66·2
Not improved	8·0	15·9	6·0

* The samples varied slightly in size. See p. 125 *n.* 1.

compared to a quarter at Moordale, and only one-sixteenth at Northtown.

The figures for 'Financial Status' (4) bear out the previous comment about Health Service patients at Crown Lodge. They represent over a third of patients discharged, though only a tenth of the standing population.

There is no clear-cut correlation between fee-paying and occupational class. This is to be expected, since occupational class, as set out here, is not directly related to income but to social responsibility.

The overwhelming majority of patients discharged are voluntary patients (5), although each hospital has in the standing population a fair proportion of certified patients (Crown Lodge 27·6 per cent, Moordale 23·3 per cent. Northtown has a very high proportion, 79·8 per cent). This confirms the picture of each hospital as 'two hospitals'—one largely static, and the other with a rapid turnover.

The possible variation of standards in diagnosis (6) between one mental hospital and another is considerable (see p. 112). The similarity between the Crown Lodge and Northtown figures may therefore be purely a result of chance—and it is important to stress that diagnosis of this kind is inclined to be arbitrary, a mere label attached to a complex and individual human problem. The classification 'mixed atypical' includes personality disorders and cases which cannot easily be classified under the other two headings. It is interesting to see that Moordale has less schizophrenics and more 'mixed atypical' patients in the sample than the other two hospitals. This may reflect caution in diagnosis.

The majority of patients in the samples for all three hospitals have been discharged one week to 6 months after admission. Crown Lodge 96 per cent, Northtown 83 per cent, Moordale 85 per cent. The national average (1956) was 72·9 per cent.[1] The figures confirm the assumption (see patient-census) that a patient who has been in hospital for more than two years may be classified as 'long-stay'. Only two at Northtown and one at Moordale were discharged after that time, while

[1] This figure of course refers to all patients, and not only to first admissions.

all the discharges from Crown Lodge were in the two-year period.

It is interesting to see that, although most of Crown Lodge's patients are fee-paying, less leave the hospital 'not improved' than at Northtown, where there are no fees; but it has already been shown that these figures are not reliable, since there is no common standard between the three hospitals, or even from doctor to doctor.

Summary

An analysis of patients included in these three samples shows definite trends. In all three hospitals, patients discharged after one period of treatment are likely to have been voluntary patients, and to have been in hospital for only a few weeks. Most of them are people in middle life, probably with settled home backgrounds. They probably have a very much better chance of recovery than patients had even ten years ago, when the stay in hospital was longer and more patients went in against their will. The experience of hospital treatment then was a much more disturbing experience. In 1956–7, it caused only a minor break in the normal pattern of living for most patients.

The Crown Lodge sample is handicapped in its chances of recovery by several factors. It contains older patients, and more schizophrenics, than the other two. Patients have been in hospital for a shorter space of time. They tend to go back to forms of work involving more responsibility and mental effort. The Northtown sample is handicapped because most patients tend to go back to working-class homes, where there may be financial difficulty. The pressures to return to work quickly are stronger, though the form of work may be less stressful. Moordale, as always, presents a mixed picture; some patients are returning to the industrial slums, some to the prosperous farms and comfortable outer suburbs; there is a greater range in age, and a considerable caution in diagnosis and prognosis on discharge.

The general results obtained are given in Table 15, overleaf.

The figures for the three hospitals given in Table 15 show a surprising degree of similarity—there is no statistical significance

TABLE 15

Results of Random Sample

Position June 1959 (i.e. 2 years 3 months to 2 years 8 months after discharge)

	Crown Lodge	Northtown	Moordale
In normal employment	50·0	51·5	48·8
Still receiving psychiatric care	13·0	12·9	15·9
Readmitted to mental hospital	32·0	31·6	28·5
Died	—	—	3·0
Moved (no further information)	3·0	2·0	1·5
Not traced	2·0	2·0	2·3

NOTES:

(1) '*In normal employment.*' This criterion was preferable to 'recovered', because it avoided a qualitative judgement. In the case of a housewife who did not undertake outside employment, the phrase used in the questionnaire was 'now carrying out normal household duties'. 'Normal' employment was taken to mean employment of the kind which the patient undertook before admission to hospital—e.g. a University student who became a shop assistant, or a housewife who required substantially more help in the house than she had previously had, would not be counted as in 'normal' employment. This category included some patients who were still receiving psychiatric care. The figures are broken down in Table 16 below.

(2) '*Still receiving psychiatric care.*' This category included those who were attending an out-patient clinic; in contact with local authority Mental Health Services; or regularly consulting their general practitioners or a social work agency 'for reasons connected with his/her mental illness'. It does not include those who were still receiving psychiatric care but were in normal employment. (See Table 16.)

(3) '*Readmitted to mental hospital.*' This refers to any readmission since the original date of discharge. If a patient was found to have been readmitted to any mental hospital (not necessarily the hospital of first admission) the case was closed.

(4) '*Died.*' The Moordale sample contained a slightly higher proportion of patients discharged over the age of fifty than the other two hospitals; but two of these four patients committed suicide.

(5) '*Moved.*' This refers only to patients who were known to have moved from the area, and who could not otherwise be traced. The total of patients who actually moved after discharge should also include those who were not traced, and some who were traced to another area. (See Table 17.)

in the small differences between them. Does this mean that, no matter what kind of treatment a mental patient receives, his chance of recovery and relapse are unaltered? Or, bearing in mind the differing structures of the samples, does it mean that each hospital is doing an equally efficient job with a different type of patient? The matched sample (p. 149) throws some light on this question, though it does not provide a full answer.

TABLE 16

Breakdown of 'in normal employment'

	Crown Lodge	Northtown	Moordale
Not still receiving psychiatric care	42·0	36·7	32·3
Still receiving psychiatric care	8·0	14·8	16·5
	50·0	51·5	48·8

The Crown Lodge sample has a clear majority of patients who were found to be independent of psychiatric care when the follow-up study took place. If this is taken as the real criterion of recovery, then Crown Lodge, despite the fact that the sample was heavily weighted with schizophrenics and that the length of stay was considerably shorter than the other two hospitals, has a clear lead.

It could be argued, on the other hand, that whether a patient is receiving care two years or more after discharge reflects less on the state of the patient than on the availability of community services. Crown Lodge, as previously noted, has no social worker, and does not make a practice of referring patients to anyone except their own general practitioner.

TABLE 17

Patients who moved after Discharge

	Crown Lodge	Northtown	Moordale
Moved, but subsequently traced	5·0	1·0	7·4
Known to have moved (but not subsequently traced)	3·0	4·0	1·5
Not traced	2·0	2·0	2·3
	10·0	7·0	11·2

These patients included two who emigrated to New Zealand, one who went to Australia, and one (a Chinese) who went to China; these are all included under 'known to have moved'. It seems evident that, for some patients, a period in hospital acts as a cathartic. They may take stock of their situation, and decide on another mode of life perhaps in another country; they may have to move to find work; they may move because of a broken marriage, or local prejudice, or the need to live with a relative who can care for them. Only 5/4/3·8 per cent are out of touch with the community medical and social services. This compares favourably with an earlier survey, which gave a figure of 14 per cent,[1] and may reflect an improvement in community care between 1953–4 and 1957–9.

TABLE 18

Condition on Discharge compared with condition on Follow-up

(*a*) CROWN LODGE

	Condition on discharge:			
	Recovered	Relieved	Not Improved	Total
Condition on follow-up:				
In normal employment	24·0	23·0	3·0	50·0
Not in normal employment	8·0	4·0	1·0	13·0
Readmitted	11·0	19·0	2·0	32·0
Not traced, or moved	2·0	2·0	1·0	5·0
Total	45·0	48·0	7·0	100·0

(*b*) NORTHTOWN

	Condition on discharge:			
	Recovered	Relieved	Not Improved	Total
Condition on follow-up:				
In normal employment	23·7	20·8	7·0	51·5
Not in normal employment	9·0	3·9	—	12·9
Readmitted	5·9	18·7	7·0	31·6
Not traced, or moved	1·0	1·1	1·9	4·0
Total	39·6	44·5	15·9	100·0

[1] Jones, K., 'Mental After-care in Lancashire', *Sociological Review*, June 1954—sample of 132 patients discharged from Hospital 'C' in the first quarter of 1953.

(*c*) MOORDALE

	Condition on discharge:			
	Recovered	Relieved	Not Improved	Total
Condition on follow-up:				
In normal employment	15·7	30·8	2·3	48·8
Not in normal employment	2·3	12·9	·7	15·9
Readmitted	6·8	20·2	1·5	28·5
Not traced, or moved	2·3	1·5	—	3·8
Died	·7	·8	1·5	3·0
Total	27·8	66·2	6·0	100·0

These tables give the full breakdown from which readmission figures were selected for Table 6.

TABLE 19

Breakdown of 'receiving psychiatric care'

This refers to patients still in the care of an agency in the community by reason of their mental illness, whether in employment or not.*

	Percentage of total patient-sample		
	Crown Lodge	Northtown	Moordale
Psychiatric Out-patient Clinic	6·0	5·0	6·0
Local Authority Mental Health Dept.	—	6·0	3·0
General Practitioner	15·0	13·7	18·0
Other agency	—	3·0	5·4

* The figures overlap, since some patients were receiving more than one form of care.

'Other agency' included several patients suffering from alcoholism who were in close touch with Alcoholics Anonymous, and two in an Industrial Rehabilitation Unit. The outstanding fact emerging from this table is the person carrying most responsibility for care of discharged mental patients in the community is the general practitioner. Local authority Mental Health Departments are at present taking a much smaller part of the load—a fact which confirms the necessity for the rapid expansion of local authority services envisaged by the Mental Health Act 1959, and also the necessity for increased attempts to sensitize general practitioners to psychiatric problems. (Our attempts to obtain information from general practitioners for this survey did not dispose us to rate their interest in psychiatric community care highly; but the poor response may have been due to lack of enthusiasm for this project, not for their patients.)

The table also shows clearly the difference in practice between Crown Lodge, where referrals are made to general practitioners and the hospital runs its own private out-patient clinic, and the other two hospitals, which use social work agencies, statutory and voluntary, in addition.

Summary

The facts which emerge most clearly from the random sample results are these:

(1) It is not true that, as is so often said in the mental health field, 'they always go back'. Patients discharged from these three hospitals in 1956–7 after one period of treatment had one chance in two, or a little more, of making a complete recovery; and only one chance in three, or a little less, of a relapse within two years sufficient to send them back to hospital again.

(2) Mental health departments in these three areas do not appear to be carrying a heavy long-term case-load.

(3) Out-patient clinics similarly deal with a smaller proportion of ex-patients than might have been expected. Our contacts with out-patient clinics during the survey led us to believe that much of the work of those we were in touch with was concerned with pre-care (i.e. with those patients who were sent on to a mental hospital after one or two visits to the clinic) or with alternative care (i.e. with patients who did not enter a mental hospital at all).

(4) The general practitioner carries a relatively heavy burden.

(5) There is no difference of statistical significance in the relapse rates of the three hospitals. This could be purely fortuitous, the differences in structure between the three samples

in effect cancelling each other out. For this reason, we proceeded to consider the results of matched samples.

From the random sample, matched cases were selected for further analysis. 90 cases (i.e. 30 from each hospital) could be matched on criteria of sex, age, diagnosis and social class.[1] The criteria are those used for the random sample.

TABLE 20

Composition of Matched Sample

1. SEX		
	Male	10
	Female	20
2. AGE		
	under 20	nil
	20–29	5
	30–39	8
	40–49	8
	50–59	6
	60–69	3
	70–79	nil
	80 and over	nil
3. OCCUPATIONAL CLASS		
	Class I	3
	Class II	15
	Class III	12
4. DIAGNOSIS		
	Affective disorder	22
	Schizophrenia	7
	Mixed atypical	1

As the male sample was very small, occupational class was also used as a criterion for female patients in the sample. Where the records stated only 'Housewife', case-records were read in full, and enquiries made of hospital staff, so that a ranking could be given.

An attempt was made to match 'diagnosis' more closely than

[1] A larger sample of matched cases was attempted, but could not be obtained. See p. 194.

the table would suggest. The 'mixed atypical' patients all suffered from psychopathic disorder; and in dealing with affective disorder, we matched patients of similar duration and severity of illness as far as possible.

By comparison with the random sample, the matched sample is heavily weighted on the affective disorders, and there are comparatively few schizophrenics. There are few patients over sixty, and none over seventy. We should therefore expect the results to be rather better than those of the random sample, and this was in fact so.

TABLE 21

Comparison of Results of Matched and Random Samples (percentage)

	Matched sample (total 90 cases)	Random sample (average of 3 hospitals)
Now in normal employment	54·4	50·1
Readmitted to mental hospital	26·7	30·7

TABLE 22

Results of Matched Sample: Raw figures per hospital

	Crown Lodge	Northtown	Moordale
Now in normal employment	20	15	14
Still receiving psychiatric care	4	4	3
Readmitted to mental hospital	4	11	9
Died	nil	nil	2
Moved	nil	nil	1
Not traced	2	nil	1

The numbers are, of course, very small for a detailed breakdown, and no great reliance can be placed upon them; but they do show that the position of Crown Lodge (for which the random sample was heavily weighted with schizophrenics) is considerably improved when cases are matched.

The similarity between the figures for Northtown and Moordale is striking.

The difficulty in securing matched cases from these three hospitals arose from the fact that they take very different types of patients. Occupational class was the most difficult factor to match, since the patients discharged from Crown Lodge are mainly in Classes I and II, and those from Northtown mainly in Class III. In hospitals with similar types of patients, this method of measurement might be employed with a greater degree of success.

8. *Average costs*

Costing, in the Hospitals Service, tends to be misunderstood. Crude average costs, obtained by dividing total expenditure under broad subjective headings by some simple unit (such as the average cost of maintaining a patient for one week) are sometimes regarded as measures of efficiency. That they cannot be so regarded stems from three fundaments of their construction.

In the first instance, the clinical purposes of hospitals even of similar size and type differ. Constellations of illnesses treated and ranges of clinical services provided vary widely, and these variations have an effect on costs quite unrelated to the question of efficiency.

Secondly, the physical circumstances under which hospitals do their work differ. Age, quality, and arrangement of buildings and grounds differ from one hospital to another and, once again, these differences have their effect on costs. If cost comparisons are to be regarded as tests of efficiency, the units compared must have similar physical circumstances, and this is seldom possible in the hospitals service.

Thirdly, the selection of the cost unit is important. The average cost of maintaining a patient for one week is an appropriate unit only where total expenditure might be expected to vary directly with patient capacities. In other cases, where total expenditure might be expected to vary in relation to some other factor, another unit would be more appropriate. Thus heating costs vary according to the efficiency of the boiler plant, the cubic space to be heated, the degree of insulation of the buildings and their general arrangement, and average patient-week

TABLE 23

Total Expenditure and Average Cost per Patient-week
Year ended 31st March 1958

	Crown Lodge		Northtown		Moordale	
	Total Expend.	Average cost per Pat.-week	Total Expend.	Average cost per Pat.-week	Total Expend.	Average cost per Pat.-week
	£	£ s. d.	£	£ s. d.	£	£ s. d.
Salaries and Wages						
Medical	11,130	14 4	34,841	4 10	11,656	11 9
Professional &c.	3,959	5 1	20,441	2 10	5,979	6 0
Nursing	67,968	4 7 7	297,427	2 1 8	60,618	3 1 0
Drugs and Dressings	3,064	3 11	11,879	1 8	3,602	3 7
Medical &c. Equip.	658	10	4,388	7	557	7
Occupational Therapy	334	5	2,170	4	956	1 0
Catering	53,390	3 8 10	169,238	1 3 8	39,178	1 19 5
Laundry	7,583	9 9	17,873	2 6	5,285	5 4
Cleaning and Porters	22,317	1 8 9	24,255	3 5	11,993	12 1
Domestic Repairs &c.	9,491	12 3	14,786	2 1	4,883	4 11
Power, Light, Heat &c.	18,323	1 3 7	61,217	8 7	17,959	18 1
Maintenance of Buildings &c.	15,858	1 0 5	81,191	11 4	8,342	8 5
Maintenance of Grounds &c.	2,749	3 7	8,293	1 2	6,709	6 9
Administration	19,062	1 4 8	25,734	3 7	13,300	13 5
Other Expenses	30,301	1 19 1	82,897	11 7	16,326	16 5
Gross Cost	266,187	17 3 1	856,630	5 19 10	207,343	10 8 9
Less Direct Credits	17,221	1 2 2	23,264	3 3	16,570	16 8
Net Cost	248,966	16 0 11	833,366	5 16 7	190,773	9 12 1
Unit Costs:						
Catering (person fed/week)						
Provisions only		1 11 0		18 7		1 5 3
Total cost		2 3 7		1 2 10		1 13 0
Number of units		(447)		(2838)		(455)
Laundry (100 articles)						
Salaries and Wages		1 8 1		13 9		1 0 9
Total cost		2 0 3		19 7		1 16 9
Number of units		(3768)		(17068)		(2873)
Average number of occupied beds		298		2800		381
Percentage occupation of total beds		84·7		98·0		84·8

costs for heating reflect all these factors,[1] which might, or might not, vary in proportion to variations in patient capacities.

Average patient-week costs have their main value in relating total expenditure by a hospital to its size, and in providing an expression in financial terms of the clinical, organizational and physical differences between hospitals which have given rise to cost differentials between them. Total expenditure by the three mental hospitals, and average costs per patient-week for a year ending in 1957–8, together with some other unit costs, are shown in Table 23.

The considerable differences between the average patient-week costs recorded for the three hospitals are indicative of the differences in circumstances and methods to be found in them. To some extent, the low cost at Northtown reflects the advantage of large-scale administration, but many other factors have an impact on the figures. The main causes of cost differential revealed by inquiry proved to be:

Salaries and Wages. A major factor in the incidence of medical and nursing salaries is the proportions of short- and long-stay to total patients in the hospital. Relatively little of the doctors' time is devoted to long-stay patients at any of the hospitals, and at Northtown these patients receive less attention from the nursing staff than do short-stay patients. In consequence, the higher the proportion of long-stay to total patients, the lower is the average cost of medical and nursing care for all patients likely to be. This largely explains the relatively low cost of medical and nursing salaries per patient-week at Northtown, where the great majority of the patients are long-stay, as compared with the other two hospitals. This subject is dealt with in greater detail in Chapter VIII.

The ratio of nursing staff to patients varies as between the three hospitals: 1 : 3 at Crown Lodge; 1 : 5·25 at Northtown; 1 : 4 at Moordale, and this factor, too, contributes to the cost differences. Additionally, at Crown Lodge, proportionally more trained, and therefore more highly paid, nurses are employed than at the other two hospitals.

[1] From 1st April 1957 some hospitals have prepared departmental costs under the Ministry of Health's 'Main Scheme', and units appropriate to the activities of each separately costed department have been selected for the expression of the costs. The 'Main Scheme' does not, however, apply to mental hospitals.

Northtown enjoys some advantages of scale in the employment of professional staff, as compared with the other hospitals. It is big enough to employ people for professional and technical work full-time within the hospital, whilst Crown Lodge and Moordale are dependent on services provided by other hospitals. To some extent this factor accounts for the differences in average patient-week costs for professional, etc., salaries between the hospitals. Once again, however, the proportion of long-stay to total patients has an effect. Long-stay patients make relatively less call on the time of most professional workers (though they may make relatively greater demands on occupational therapists, whose salaries are included under this head).

Drugs and Dressings. Differences in clinical orientation affect the amount of drugs prescribed, and this is a difficult matter to give judgement on. A major factor, again, is the proportion of long-stay to total patients.

Medical and Surgical Equipment. Expenditure under this heading in the Hospitals Service tends to conceal rather than to reveal information. The cost of major capital equipment is included neither in the year of its purchase nor as an annual depreciation charge. Whilst the first of these alternatives would inflate costs in the year of development, it would at least give some idea of relative investment. Despite deficiencies in the theory and practice of depreciation accounting, the second method would provide some indication of relative use of equipment. The figure actually provided includes only minor purchases and repair and maintenance costs. It has no special significance.

The same argument applies, though because of their relative durability, with less force, to the costs shown for buildings and grounds.

Occupational Therapy. Costs shown under this heading refer to equipment and materials only.

Catering. Patient-week costs for catering are especially misleading, since the hospital additionally feeds most of its staff, and the ratio of staff to patients varies from one hospital to another. A separate unit cost is provided at the foot of Table 23 showing cost in terms of one person fed for one week. The figures confirm our observation that the standard of food supplied at Crown Lodge is higher than at the other two hospitals. All three hospitals have bulk buying arrangements for provisions: Crown Lodge through the agency of a commercial catering concern, Northtown having a joint contracting committee with another hospital, and Moordale participating in a group purchasing scheme.

Laundry. For similar reasons, a separate unit cost is provided for laundry services at the foot of Table 23. Two factors affect the operative effectiveness of the laundry service: the unit cost of operating the laundry, and the frequency with which laundry service is supplied to the wards and departments. The first factor is described by the unit cost per 100 articles laundered. In this respect, Northtown enjoys an advantage of scale. It is big enough to employ at full capacity a specialized laundry service, and the resulting unit cost is approximately only one-half of the costs returned by the smaller hospitals. The intensity of the laundry service can be indicated by dividing the number of units laundered in each hospital by its population (both figures are given in Table 23). The results of this calculation are:

TABLE 24

Average Number of Garments Laundered per Patient per annum

Crown Lodge	Northtown	Moordale
1,264	609	754

One might therefore assume that the higher cost per patient-week of the laundry service at Crown Lodge results from (*a*) the high cost of running a small laundry, and (*b*) rapid turnover of linen. Conversely, the low cost at Northtown stems from (*a*) the low cost of large-scale laundry operations and (*b*) relatively less frequent changes of linen. Moordale's figure reflects, operating in opposite directions, (*a*) high costs of a small laundry, and (*b*) changes of linen less frequently than at Crown Lodge.

Cleaning and Portering. These figures show in sharp relief differences in practice at the three hospitals. At Crown Lodge patients, nearly all of whom are fee-paying, do not carry out utility work in the hospital, and the cost of cleaning and porterage is £1 8*s*. 9*d*. per patient-week. At Northtown, most utility work is done by the patients, and the cost of the remaining work, which is done by outside workers, is 3*s*. 5*d*. per patient-week. At Moordale some work is done by patients, but much is not, and the cost of external employees falls between the other two hospitals at 12*s*. 1*d*. per week.

Perhaps more clearly than any of the other costs, the cleaning and portering figures illustrate that average patient-week costs do not directly operate as indices of efficiency. The employment of patients in utility work might be occasioned because the work is considered clinically desirable for them. Or it might arise simply because there is no one else available to do the work. Whichever reason applies, the effect on the cost is the same: the more patient labour used, the less the cost will be.

Domestic Repairs, Maintenance of Buildings and Grounds. Here, the same considerations apply. Patient-labour is used extensively on repair and maintenance work at Northtown, to some extent at Moordale, and very little at Crown Lodge, though the 'activity groups' for long-stay patients which are described in Chapter II do a little work. Patient labour is paid at very low rates, but working hours are short, usually three to five hours per day, and the pace of work is slow.

Maintenance work at Moordale, which was constructed in 1902, is frequently less pressing than that at Crown Lodge, which was built in 1850, and at Northtown, 1852. Buildings do not improve as they grow older, and higher maintenance costs might be expected at Northtown and Crown Lodge. Maintenance, however, is not merely a matter of doing the jobs which are necessary to preserve the fabric of the buildings. At Crown Lodge a high standard of furnishing and décor is maintained throughout the hospital, and the high figures shown for upkeep reflect the results achieved. The lower figures for Northtown and Moordale are descriptive of the lower standards which financial considerations have enforced on those hospitals.

Power, Light and Heat. Costs under this head depend partly on the standard of the service provided and partly on the physical circumstances under which it is provided. To some extent the high cost at Crown Lodge reflects the provision of special amenities, for instance coal fires are provided for some patients all the year round, and this is not the case at Northtown and Moordale.

Once again, Northtown has the advantage of size in heating costs in particular. Bigger heating installations are generally capable of operating at lower cost per unit of heat provided than are smaller ones.

Administration. Under this heading are included the salaries of administrative staff in secretarial, financial and medical records departments, and administrative equipment, etc. The high figure at Crown Lodge reflects the private status of the hospital outside the National Health Service. One of the disadvantages of independent status is the necessity to provide all necessary administrative services without assistance from an outside agency, such as a Regional Hospital Board.[1] Northtown's low figure again reflects an advantage of scale. Administrative responsibility, particularly in finance departments, does not increase in proportion to patient populations: it is not more difficult to pay for provisions for one thousand patients than it is to pay for five hundred, and it is sometimes easier to arrange a wages routine for a staff of five hundred than it is to pay one hundred. Again, the question is not merely one of efficiency. The costs are a reflection of status and size differences and of administrative arrangements.

Other Expenses. This heading covers a multitude of miscellaneous expenses not capable of analysis under the main headings. The figure for Crown Lodge includes some costs which would not be applicable to the other hospitals, for example, insurances, the cost of running private cars for the use of patients, and the maintenance of private consulting rooms in a nearby city. In the year in question the figure was unduly inflated by a payment of arrears of rates following the settlement of a rating claim in favour of the local authority.

The multitude of influences which affect average patient-week

[1] In some regions, primary accounting functions, for example the preparation of wages and stores records and the analysis of costs, have been centralized. This procedure enables much manual accounting to be superseded by machine installations and the saving in cost may be considerable.

costs, which have been described, sufficiently support the contention that such figures cannot be regarded as indices of efficiency. Perhaps their most useful function is to show where important differences in clinical method, staffing, administration or physical circumstances exist between hospitals, as a stimulus to further enquiry.

VIII

COMPLEX MEASURES OF EFFICIENCY

A COMPLEX measure of efficiency involves the use of two or more simple measures in combination to provide a more adequate index of work done. There are three basic problems in the construction of such a measure: the selection of the factors to be measured, the method of combination, and the allocation of weights.

1. *Selection.* The simple measures selected must be meaningful in themselves, and capable of being brought into relationship with each other.

2. *Combination.* They must be so combined as to provide checks and balances, one remedying the deficiency of another as far as possible.

3. *Weighting.* If several simple measures are involved, they may not be of equal value or importance. Judgement is involved in allotting a due weight to each factor, so that the final measure is a balanced one.

Qualitative Measures

A study of the Visitors' Books of early county asylums makes it evident that, even in the first half of the nineteenth century, visiting justices and commissioners used a rudimentary qualitative approach to efficiency. The repetition of such entries as 'Patients quiet—all very clean and comfortable' or 'The patients are well cared for, and the covers neatly arranged on the beds during the day' show that the official visitors had clear, if very limited, ideas of what they were looking for. 'Lunatics' were by nature noisy, violent, disorganized and dirty. The visitors looked therefore for quietness, tractability, order and cleanliness, and do not seem to have enquired closely whether these desirable results were brought about by intimidation, or large overdoses of croton oil, as they sometimes were.

In 1827, a group of parliamentary reformers, led by Lord Ashley,[1] published a series of 'Inquiries Relative to Lunatic Asylums and the Treatment of the Insane'. These were sent, in the form of a questionnaire, to medical superintendents of asylums, though the group had no power to compel the making of a return.

This questionnaire is the earliest example of an attempt to obtain a controlled judgement of the relative efficiency of asylums. An emphasis on cleanliness and basic hygiene was to be expected; but the questionnaire also contained searching enquiries into methods of patient-management:

> How far has manual labour been adopted with advantage, and with what description of patients?
>
> . . . has benefit been experienced by furnishing the patients in their courtyards with means of innocent amusement, from music, domestic animals, poultry, birds, flowers, and objects of a similar nature?
>
> Is it the opinion of the superintendent that a state of entire indolence and mental inertness is decidedly prejudicial to the patient?

This approach through questions which demand answers in the form of value-judgements does not seem to have been widely used again in England; but it has been used again in recent years in the United States. In 1953, the Committee on Hospitals of the American Group for the Advancement of Psychiatry published an 'Outline to be used as a Guide to the Evaluation of Treatment in a Public Psychiatric Hospital'. Though much more complex, and framed in a different context, this uses the same basic approach as the English questionnaire of 1827; and an examination of the questions asked may illustrate some of the dangers of the qualitative method.

[1] Later the seventh Earl of Shaftesbury, and Chairman of the Lunacy Commission for many years.

The American questionnaire contains 315 separate questions, covering a wide range of hospital activities, from 'Food' to 'Family Care', and from 'Recreation' to 'Research'. These questions fall into three categories. Some can be answered unequivocally 'Yes' or 'No', e.g.:

13. Do patients and employees receive the same standard menu?
84. Are there two sheets to each bed?
274. Is there a consultant in tuberculosis?

Others require a little statistical work, though the basis on which figures are suggested is not made clear:

134. Is there one qualified and licensed dentist for each 1,000 patients?
206. Is the autopsy percentage above 20 per cent?
301. Are assistants in occupational therapy available in a ratio of
    (*a*) 1 : 150 patients on the chronic service?
    (*b*) 1 : 140 on the acute service?

There is no indication of why an occupational therapist should be able to handle ten less short-stay patients than long-stay patients, or whether a high percentage of autopsies is commendable or not.

A third type of question involves the exercise of considerable personal judgement:

2. Is the superintendent . . . given authority *commensurate with his responsibility*?
168. Is there *an adequate programme* of recreation?
203. Is there *a properly equipped* laboratory?
217. Are there *a sufficient number* of electric shock units?

No valid comparisons can be made on the grounds of different medical superintendents' estimates of whether they possess 'commensurate' authority; or of what they consider 'adequate' recreation for patients; or of what they judge to be the 'proper' equipment for a laboratory; or of how many electric shock units they consider 'sufficient'. (In this last instance, a psychoanalytically orientated psychiatrist might consider one a superfluity.)

From a research point of view, therefore, the answers to these questions will be of very unequal value.

The proportioning of the questionnaire reveals some anomalies. Out of 315 questions, 24 deal with catering and kitchen management, but only eight with 'Hospital and Community', seven with 'Training and Research', and two with 'Family Care'. 'Are voluntary admissions encouraged?' (243) takes up no more space than 'Are personal deodorants available?' (103).

No indication is given of the relative importance of individual enquiries. An outside observer might be forgiven if he drew the conclusion from this questionnaire that mechanical dishwashers (three questions) were more important than case-histories (one question), or that personal deodorants were the therapeutic equivalent of personal liberty.

To be fair, it is nowhere suggested that the answer to every question should have equal weight; but neither is an indication given of the relative weightings to be employed. The prevalence of this type of questionnaire in American life is such that some psychiatrists may well be likely to add up the number of 'right answers'—and to draw very wrong conclusions from them.

The committee responsible for drawing up the questionnaire states rightly in the prefatory notes that it may serve 'as a reminder of the complex nature of hospital operations, and as a guide and help in their continued improvement'. They are on less sure ground when they suggest that it 'not only serves as one means of gauging staff achievement, but helps in the evaluation of specific aspects of the hospital programme'. A questionnaire of this type cannot 'gauge' or 'evaluate'. It can only suggest factors to be kept in mind.

Measures of this type are inherently biased. The selection of factors, by some common agreement as to what is 'important', is not a fully rational process. There is still an emphasis on details of domestic management—not necessarily because this is now more 'important' than medical or social factors in treatment, but because it is easier to deal with in a question-and-answer manner. It is not difficult to make a list of 24 questions concerned with food and kitchen equipment where commonly-accepted standards apply, at any rate within a given culture. It would be much more difficult to think of 24 meaningful questions about medical treatment or social care, and impossible to do so without laying down rigid principles incapable of universal application.

In this measure, the combination of factors is not even attempted—each question stands alone; and there is no weighting. The mixture of qualitative and quantitative questions evokes a mixture of subjective and objective answers without indicating that these may have different values. Questionnaires of this type may have a limited value in spurring individual hospital administrators, medical or lay, to action; but they can give rise to some misleading assumptions, and are of little or no value for comparisons of working efficiency.

Quantitative Measures: the W.H.O. measures

A few months after the publication of the American 'Outline', the World Health Organization's Expert Committee published a scheme of a very different kind.[1] This consisted of five different measures: length of stay, admission and discharge, admission and beddage, average cost, and relapse rate. The main recommendations for the refinement of these five measures are set down below:

(*a*) *Length of stay.* The average length of stay should be determined separately for three groups of patients: those discharged in less than a year; those discharged between one and five years after admission; and those 'who stay more than five years, and in most cases never leave the hospital'. The optimal period of discharge for the first group was thought to be about two to three months, and for the second group, about eighteen months. If these periods were passed, patients tended to move from one category to another.

(*b*) *The relation between admission and discharge rates* was to be measured by the ratio between the number of patients admitted to a given number of beds, and the numbers discharged 'cured' or 'improved' from those beds. This refines the discharge statistics considerably by cutting out those discharged 'not improved' from the calculation, and by making separate calculations for different classes of patients.

(*c*) *The capacity of absorption* was to be calculated by dividing the admission rate by the total beddage, the 'index of absorption' being:

$$\frac{100 \text{ patients admitted}}{100 \text{ beds}} = 1.$$

[1] Third Report of Expert Committee on Mental Health, September 1953.

It was added that this index would enable comparisons to be made between hospitals dealing with the same types of patient.

(*d*) *Average cost* was to be measured in terms of the cost of the average stay in hospital rather than in terms of the cost per day or per week.

$$\text{Average length of stay} \times \text{cost per day} = \text{average cost.}$$

This introduces a valuable new concept: that of *cost per case* rather than cost for a specified period of time.

(*e*) *Ratio between patients relapsed and discharged.* This was to be based on the proportion of patients readmitted to hospital within a pre-determined period—two or five years being suggested.

The W.H.O. measures have a number of points in their favour. They are simple to operate, and clear-cut. They are purely quantitative, and thus free from value-judgements. They are relatively free from cultural limitations. The selection is sound, because only a few factors are involved, and these are all directly concerned with the progress of patients.

The Committee wisely did not claim to have produced an exhaustive measure, but merely to have set out some of the factors 'which help assess the value of a mental hospital'.

For these reasons, the W.H.O. measures were taken as the starting-point of our attempt to find a means of assessing the relative efficiency of Crown Lodge, Northtown and Moordale. They were, however, taken with reservations; for while the measures were suitable on the grounds of selection, they were not capable of combination, and no indication was given of the weight to be attached to each. The W.H.O. Committee had produced five useful and valuable criteria, but these did not add up to a complex measure of efficiency.

When we tried to apply these measures to the three hospitals, certain other grounds for criticism became apparent:

1. The relation between admission and discharge rates was dependent on individual psychiatrists' judgements of whether their patients were 'cured' or 'improved' at the time of discharge. We had found that such judgements were largely unrelated to the pattern of subsequent admission (see p. 125).

2. The capacity of absorption could only be used for hospitals dealing with the same types of patient. We had established by

means of the patient-census that Crown Lodge, Northtown and Moordale dealt with very different types of patient.

3. The length of stay was listed separately from the cost per case; but in fact length of stay was taken into account in computing cost per case, and it seemed unnecessary to include this factor twice.

For these reasons, we decided to abandon for practical purposes measurement of the relation between admission and discharge rates, the capacity of absorption, and the length of stay. This left cost per case—in itself a complex measure, since it includes both the cost of treatment and the duration of treatment; and the relapse rate.

These two factors appeared in themselves to offer a useful approach to the question of a measure of efficiency. The use of cost as a basis for such a measure has two arguments to commend it. First, it enables the common measure of money to be applied to all the heterogeneous activities of the hospitals compared. Tests of other types are at best piecemeal, for they focus attention on one feature of hospital activity to the exclusion of all others. Cost accounting resolves all activities to a single standard, monetary cost. Second, costing gives due weight to differences in physical resources between hospitals, reflecting the high level of expense required to maintain well-equipped and fully-staffed hospitals in relation to those less favourably placed.

Patient-week costs, as shown in Chapter 7, are not in themselves an adequate measure; but cost per case, as defined by the W.H.O. Committee, took into account not only the daily or weekly average cost, but also the length of time which the treatment of individual patients took. Other factors being equal, it is clearly more efficient to treat a patient at a cost of £20 a week for four weeks than to treat him at a cost of £5 a week for six months.

The major source of bias in such a calculation lies in the subsequent relapse rate. If the majority of patients treated for four weeks are readmitted to hospital, and the majority of patients treated for six months are not, the latter may prove more efficient in the long run.

We therefore proceeded to carry out a detailed investigation of cost per case in the three hospitals, the question of the relapse rate being kept in mind as a possible weighting factor.

IX

COST PER CASE

THE device of cost per case, as suggested by the World Health Organization's Expert Committee, is deceptively simple. The calculation 'average length of stay × cost per day' (or per week) confuses two different types of measurement. Average patient-week costs are calculated by taking total expenditure on all patients, and dividing by total occupied beddage. The resulting statistics are a reflection of the cost of maintaining all patients, short-stay and long-stay alike. Average length of stay, on the other hand, can only be computed for patients who have been discharged. In any given period, the overwhelming majority of patients discharged will be short-stay patients.

A pilot survey of three hospitals by Wadsworth, Tonge and Barber (1957)[1] attempted refinements of the W.H.O. measure. It was not possible to separate short-stay and long-stay costs entirely, since these overlapped in so many ways; but the costs of three major factors in treatment—medical care, nursing care, and drugs and dressings—could be so separated. The cost of these three factors only was computed for selected short-stay wards, and was multiplied by the average length of stay for patients discharged from those wards. In addition, patients' loss of earnings during hospitalization were computed at a flat rate of £8 per week, and this sum was added to the cost per case in an attempt to show the 'total cost of mental illness'.

On this basis, it could be shown that the hospital with the highest patient-week costs actually had the lowest cost per case,

[1] W. V. Wadsworth, W. L. Tonge and L. E. Barber, 'The Cost and Efficiency of Mental Hospitals', *Lancet*, September 1957.

because patients were restored to the community more quickly.

This measure was valuable in that it overcame the difficulty of confusing long-stay and short-stay costs by narrowing the calculation to short-stay wards only; and it excluded many extraneous factors (such as the age and quality of hospital buildings) which cause cost differentials. It concentrated on three factors where fairly strict comparison was possible; medical salaries, nursing salaries, and pharmaceutical costs.

The introduction of a weighting for loss of earnings, however, was open to objection for two reasons. Mental patients, like any other vertical class in the community, have a varied earning power. To compute loss of earnings for a company director and an unskilled labourer equally at £8 a week is meaningless. Moreover, the 'total cost of mental illness', if it could be assessed, would have to include many other factors, such as the cost of community services before and after hospitalization, the cost of sick benefit, and incidental costs to the patient's family.

In spite of this weakness, the Wadsworth, Tonge and Barber survey had introduced a useful refinement into the calculation. Cost per case figures could be computed if three conditions were satisfied:

(1) The costing was restricted to factors for which reliable separate costs for long-stay and short-stay wards are calculable.

(2) Cost per case referred only to short-stay cost per week × length of stay. It would be possible, of course, to compute a cost per case for long-stay patients also. If the present trend to activate such patients, and to return them to the community continues, it may soon be possible to work out a separate length of stay for such patients. At present, however, as the World Health Organization report noted, the chances of a patient being discharged after more than five years in hospital are very small indeed, and the only basis for a cost per case calculation would be long-stay cost per week × expectation of life. It would be difficult to assess the value of this calculation, since the hospital with the highest long-stay cost might well be the most efficient—because it kept its patients alive longer. For these reasons, present calculations have been restricted to short-stay patients.

Short-stay cost per week

Calculations on the lines indicated above are undertaken for Crown Lodge, Northtown and Moordale, with the following results:

TABLE 25

Medical Staff Salaries: Cost per Patient-week

	Crown Lodge £ *s.* *d.*	Northtown £ *s.* *d.*	Moordale £ *s.* *d.*
Clinical care of			
short-stay patients	17.8	7.6	13.11
long-stay patients	4.3	1.6	3. 5
Other duties	3.9	1.5	2. 7

NOTES:

(1) These costs are based on records of employment of doctors' time during a test month in the spring of 1959. See Table 10.

(2) The allocation of time, when applied to gross salaries payable during the test month, provide the proportions of total medical salaries cost applicable to each of the categories tabulated above. The average patient-week costs are calculated by applying these proportions to the total medical salaries cost for 1957–8 shown in Table 23, i.e.

$$\text{Total cost of medical salaries 1957–8} \times \frac{\text{Prop. of cost in test month}}{\text{Total cost in test month}} \times \frac{7}{365} \times \frac{1}{n}$$

(3) For the clinical care of long-stay and short-stay patients, $n =$ the average number of patients in each category. For other duties, $n =$ the total number of patients at each hospital.

(4) As in the case of Table 11, time spent 'on call' is ignored.

(5) 'Other duties' consists of time spent on general administration, at staff- and patient-meetings, and miscellaneous.

The cost of medical clinical care is very much lower for long-stay than for short-stay patients in all three hospitals. This is what we should expect from our observations in Chapter VI, and from Table 12. Cost, however, is a reflection not only of the allocation of time, but also, since some doctors receive higher salaries than others, of the grade of staff employed. In terms of cost, for instance, five minutes with a consultant would be equivalent to rather more than fifteen minutes with a registrar.

Table 26 shows that the cost of nursing care for a long-stay patient is higher than for a short-stay patient at Crown Lodge. As we have shown in Table 5, the hospital has a high proportion

TABLE 26

Salaries and Wages of Nursing Staff: Cost per Patient-week

	Crown Lodge	Northtown	Moordale
	£ s. d.	£ s. d.	£ s. d.
Clinical care of			
short-stay patients	2. 6.11	3. 3.8	3. 8.10
long-stay patients	2.14.10	1.12.8	1. 5. 5
Other duties	1.16. 3	2.6	1. 1. 3

NOTE:

These figures are based on records kept by each hospital of the employment of their nursing staffs during a test month in the spring of 1959, and have been calculated in a similar manner to those in Table 25.

of geriatric patients (38·4 per cent of all patients being over 70) which means that there is a good deal of intensive sick-nursing. Short-stay patients attend occupational therapy or discussion-groups, and commonly spend their afternoons in the hall or canteen. For these activities, few nurses are required to be in attendance. It is quite common at Crown Lodge to find a sister or charge nurse alone in a short-stay ward during the hours of activity. The patients are all elsewhere, and more staff would be unnecessary.

At Northtown, only 12·1 per cent of patients fall in the over 70 group, so that the nursing needs for long-stay patients are less.

At Moordale, the cost of nursing care concentrates heavily on short-stay patients. As Table 12 shows, however, long-stay patients receive a higher proportion of doctors' time than at the other two hospitals. Additionally, as mentioned in Chapter IV, five social therapists are employed at Moordale. They devote much of their time to activity groups with long-stay patients, thus reducing the need for nursing staff. The employment of social therapists illustrates the difficulty of providing strictly comparable cost figures even in so restricted a field as that chosen for the survey. Differences in cost may often result from local variations in practice.

The results of the analysis of drugs and dressings are shown overleaf.

These figures were compiled from records kept by the pharmacists concerned, since they alone had the material for

TABLE 27

Analysis of Drugs, etc., used in Terms of Cost per Patient-week

Crown Lodge		Northtown		Moordale	
Short-stay	Long-stay	Short-stay	Long-stay	Short-stay	Long-stay
d.	*d.*	*d.*	*d.*	*d.*	*d.*
47·05	47·56	26·22	18·07	91·44	19·55

analysis to hand, and the capacity to interpret it. The returns showed interesting differences in medical practice with regard to the prescription of drugs. Comment on these differences is, however, beyond the field of the present authors.

Tables 25 to 27 are summarized in Table 28 below. Costs of medical and nursing time not directly allocable to either category of patient, for example time spent at meetings or on administrative work, have been apportioned equally among all patients, there being no evidence that they contributed more to the welfare of one class of patient than another.

TABLE 28

Summary of Patient-week Costs

	Crown Lodge		Northtown		Moordale	
	Short-stay	Long-stay	Short-stay	Long-stay	Short-stay	Long-stay
	£ *s.* *d.*	£ *s.* *d.*	£ *s.* *d.*	£ *s.* *d.*	£ *s.* *d.*	£ *s.* *d.*
Medical Salaries:						
clinical	17. 8	4. 3	7. 6	1. 6	13.11	3. 5
other	3. 9	3. 9	1. 5	1. 5	2. 7	2. 7
Nursing Salaries:						
clinical	2. 6.11	2.14.10	3. 3. 8	1.12. 8	3. 8.10	1. 5. 5
other	1.16. 3	1.16. 3	2. 6	2. 6	1. 1. 3	1. 1. 3
Drugs, etc.	3. 11	4. 0	2. 2	1. 6	7. 7	1. 8
Total of separately costed items	5. 8. 6	5. 3. 1	3.17. 3	1.19. 7	5.14. 2	2.14. 4

Table 28 reveals striking differences in the costs of ward treatment for long-stay and short-stay patients, of varying degrees at each hospital. In particular, they illustrate the ineffectiveness of the overall average cost per patient-week figures or ward costs, as shown in Table 23 in Chapter VII. For the costed elements, the overall averages are: Crown Lodge, £5 6*s*. 10*d*.; Northtown, £2 8*s*. 2*d*.; Moordale, £3 16*s*. 4*d*. In each case, as might be expected, the figures for short-stay patients are higher, and those for long-stay patients lower, than the general average. What the general average will be, however, clearly depends not only on the range and quality of the services provided, but also on the relative numbers of short-stay and long-stay patients treated.

Cost per case

Table 28 provides a 'short-stay patient-week cost' for the selected items. Table 13 has shown the average length of stay for a random sample of first admissions. If the two figures are multiplied together, the result is a 'cost per case' figure for first admissions—the only patients for whom the results of treatment can be measured, since they have not previously entered mental hospital.

At this point, it is necessary to consider whether a weighting factor should be introduced to express variations in the relapse rate. There are circumstances in which this would be necessary. For instance, if 25 per cent of first admissions relapsed after discharge from Hospital A. and 50 per cent after discharge from Hospital B., this would have an obvious bearing on their respective costs. Mathematically, the calculation would take the form of multiplying the cost per case by the inverse probability of recovery:

$$\text{At Hospital A.: cost per case} \times \frac{100}{75}$$

$$\text{At Hospital B.: cost per case} \times \frac{100}{50}$$

At Crown Lodge, Northtown and Moordale, however, no such variation was observed in the random sample. The differences in the relapse rates of the three hospitals were so slight that no statistical significance could be attached to them. Though the results of the matched sample have been reproduced in Chapter VII, these are so small that no great weight can be attached to them, though reference will be made to them later.

It was therefore decided to treat the probability of relapse as a constant.

The figures could have been refined in another way by restricting length-of-stay figures. A few patients discharge themselves after two or three days in hospital, and there is a good case for disregarding those whose length of stay is less than a fortnight on the grounds that they have not been in hospital long enough to receive active treatment. At the other end of the scale, there are a few patients who are discharged after several years in hospital, either because of an improvement in the home situation, or because they have successfully undergone a course of rehabilitation. If the calculation is to be confined to short-stay patients, it might be more accurate if it were restricted to those patients discharged after a stay in hospital of two weeks to two years.

In the case of the three hospitals described here, this limitation makes only a difference of a penny or two to the final figures, and is therefore omitted. The final calculation is confined to cost per short-stay patient-week × average length of stay for first admissions. This 'short-stay cost per case' figure for the separately costed items is given below, the average patient-week cost as used by the Ministry of Health being repeated for comparison:

TABLE 29

Short-stay Cost per Case

	Crown Lodge	Northtown	Moordale
(i) average cost per short-stay patient-week (separately costed items only)	£5 8*s*. 6*d*.	£3 17*s*. 3*d*.	£5 14*s*. 2*d*.
(ii) average length of stay (in days)	69·3	116·8	102·0
(iii) *Short-stay cost per case* (i) × $\frac{\text{(ii)}}{7}$	£53 14*s*. 2*d*.	£64 9*s*. 2*d*.	£83 3*s*. 7*d*.
compared with			
(iv) average patient-week cost	£16 0*s*. 11*d*.	£5 16*s*. 7*d*.	£9 12*s*. 1*d*.

It will be seen that the 'short-stay cost per case' calculation gives a very different picture of costs from the average patient-week calculation. Though the average patient-week cost at Crown Lodge is much higher than that at the other two hospitals, the clinical cost per case for first admissions is lower, largely because the average length of stay is shorter; and this result is obtained without the corollary of a higher relapse rate. In fact, the small matched sample provides supplementary evidence to show that the true relapse rate may be considerably lower at Crown Lodge than at Northtown.

It is thus cheaper, in terms of the most realistic costing measure which we have been able to devise, for a patient admitted to mental hospital for the first time to be treated at Crown Lodge than to be treated at Northtown or Moordale. As we have shown, there are many contributory factors; but we think that low cost per case at Crown Lodge is mainly due to the concentration of medical clinical effort. High cost per case at Northtown is mainly due to difficulties of organization, and the fact that the neurosis unit is not working at full efficiency. Moordale's high cost per case figure is mainly due to four factors: it is in fact, though not in name, a teaching hospital, and teaching hospital costs are normally much higher than those of other hospitals; membership of a mixed hospital group leads to diffusion of authority, which is not conducive to efficiency; drug costs are artificially inflated by the habit of dispensing for out-patients from ward stocks; and the average length of stay (102·0 days), though shorter than Northtown's 116·8, is very much greater than Crown Lodge's 69·3.

At Crown Lodge, treatment is expensive for most patients. The few Health Service patients may be aware that their length of stay is limited to six months, and therefore be anxious to secure early discharge in order to avoid transfer to another and less pleasant hospital.

We do not intend to range Crown Lodge, Northtown and Moordale in some sort of efficiency league table, with the winner at the top. We have made it plain in Chapter V that needs and resources differ too greatly for strict comparisons to be made.

PART FOUR

The Mental Hospital and the Future

X

GENERAL CONCLUSIONS

SOME years ago, a review of a book written by a social scientist ended with the comment, 'If Mr. A. has not provided the answers to the major questions which could be asked on this subject, at least he has defined the questions a little more clearly.' Perhaps the same could be said of this survey. It has raised far more questions than it has been able to answer; but we hope that in raising them, and in demonstrating some of the fallacies inherent in dogmatic answers, we have provided a beginning to the study of a very large subject.

It is no more than a beginning. We have not 'proved' (as one or two of our more enthusiastic colleagues have suggested) that 'high-cost hospitals really run more cheaply than low-cost hospitals', or that 'private enterprise is more efficient than a nationalized Health Service'. All that we have done is to subject the work of three mental hospitals first to qualitative and then to quantitative analysis, with the intention of finding clues to the concept of efficiency. No wide general conclusions can be drawn from a very limited survey.

For these reasons, we present our conclusions not in the form of dogmatic answers, but as a series of questions on which we are prepared in the main only to make tentative comments.

1. *Is there a perfect measure of efficiency for the work of mental hospitals?* We have not been able to find one. To seek such a measure is to demand that the part shall be fully and truly representative of the whole.

It may be possible in industry to measure the efficiency of an undertaking by its output or its net profits. In dealing with human groups, aims are so diversified and material is so uneven that no measure seems to be more than a rough and arbitrary guide. Some measures are less misleading than others; but none can fully measure the work of such a complex organization as a modern mental hospital.

2. *Is short-stay cost per case an improvement on existing methods of assessment?* It has been demonstrated that the average patient-week cost bears no relation to the real cost of treatment, since it takes no account of the proportions of long-stay and short-stay patients in the hospital, the way in which resources are allocated between them, or the length of treatment. The World Health Organization's proposals take the last of these factors into account, but not the other two; and the proposals are too diversified to produce a practicable measure, though they are valuable in other ways. Short-stay cost per case takes all three factors into account. It has the merit of selecting two essential sets of data—clinical costs, and the length of stay. It brings them together in a single calculation which needs no weighting, provided that the relapse rate is constant between the hospitals concerned.

This is inevitably a measure of limited scope. It describes the effectiveness of one part only of the hospitals—the wards—in relation to one class only of patients—short-stay patients.

It is not suggested by the limitation of the measure to ward costs that these, and only these, contribute to the chances of recovery of short-stay patients. Other factors, such as social work, occupational therapy, and facilities for recreation also play a part; but it is the essence of the cost per case measure that it compares the common work of all mental hospitals—the positive endeavour of doctors and nurses to improve the condition of their patients. Extension of the measure to include diverse factors would introduce complexities of accounting, and impair its general validity as a comparison on a common base.

To recapitulate, the use of the measure involves:

(i) separate calculation of short-stay costs in at least three major factors in treatment: medical salaries, nursing salaries and pharmaceutical costs. Division of the average weekly cost thus obtained by the number of short-stay beds in occupation at the hospital.

(ii) calculation of the average length of stay for patients discharged in a given period after one admission to hospital. Cases of known organic origin to be disregarded.

(iii) multiplication of (i) by (ii).

3. *Is there a satisfactory method of assessing the efficiency of the care of long-stay patients in terms of cost?* In the absence of any generally acceptable test of the well-being of long-stay patients, accounting methods can say no more than that, other things being equal, the greater amount of resources devoted to their care, the more comfortable they should be.

Splitting long-stay and short-stay clinical costs provides a check on whether a reasonable amount of the hospital's resources is being devoted to their care.

4. *Can short-stay cost per case be used for comparisons between different types of psychiatric provision?* Though the measure has been tried only on the short-stay wards of mental hospitals, there is no reason why it should not be applied to short-stay wards of psychiatric units in general hospitals.

It might also be possible to adapt it to the use of day hospitals and out-patient clinics. There are difficulties here in interpreting 'length of stay', and in eliminating the effects of other kinds of psychiatric assistance which may be given concurrently, but these are probably not insuperable. As diverse forms of care develop, comparisons in efficiency between them should throw some light on their value.

5. *Can length of stay be substantially reduced by an increase of medical clinical time?* Prima facie, it seems reasonable to answer in the affirmative. If medical treatment has a value in mental disorder (and we assume that it has) a patient who sees his doctor for two or three hours a week ought to recover more quickly than if he saw him for only a few minutes. No doubt the law of diminishing returns would apply at some point, but it is doubtful whether any mental hospital in this country has reached it yet.

However, this is an over-simplification. Dr. A. may achieve more in ten minutes with Patient B. than Dr. C. can achieve in several hours with Patient D. This may depend on the psychiatrist's own ability, the nature of the patient's illness, the stage in the course of treatment, the degree of co-operation offered by the patient, and the method of treatment employed. Thus the original question splinters into unanswerable fragments. We never get quite the same human situation twice over.

A correlation between the amount of medical clinical time devoted to short-stay patients in Crown Lodge, Northtown and Moordale (Table 12) and the length of stay (Table 13) must be treated with extreme caution, not only for the reasons which have been given, but because medical clinical time is only one factor among many in in-patient treatment. Moreover, both sets of figures are averages with large standard deviations; but they do produce a striking negative correlation ($r = -0{\cdot}9916$) which may be taken to indicate that there is some connection between intensive medical treatment and early discharge.

6. *Do improvements in staff communication lead demonstrably to greater efficiency?* The evidence from the survey is mainly negative. We have been able to show that in some cases lack of communication causes inefficiency, as in the partial isolation of the psychologists at Northtown, and the difficulties of the catering officer at Moordale. Experience at Crown Lodge suggests that the formation of formal staff groups for discussion and the communication of ideas may initially be met with some suspicion, but that this can be overcome in time, given a clear lead from the top and a certain amount of goodwill.

To set up such groups involves the exercise of authority. Genuine two-way communication (up the hierarchy as well as down from on high) is difficult to achieve, and paradoxically involves abdication from authority. Some psychiatrists may not be able to perform this piece of administrative acrobatics well; but it is unlikely that a leader without some intensive training in human relations would be able to perform it at all. A great deal depends on the personality of the person who calls the group into being, and on the way in which it is presented to members.

7. *Is the therapeutic community system of value to patients?* The principle behind this system, as practised at Crown Lodge, is that it helps the patient to identify with the hospital group, and gives him an opportunity of exercising a limited responsibility in a hospital setting. It may be questioned whether, as the length of stay becomes shorter and patient turnover increases, this is possible for the short-stay patient.

Few long-stay patients are sufficiently articulate, or sufficiently in touch with events around them, to participate in this kind of verbal expression. For those who are, it may be a valuable approach, but for most, activity groups provide a better means of socialization.

Assuming that a proportion of short-stay patients are in hospital long enough to make the system worth while, we may further question whether they should be encouraged to identify with the hospital group, or whether attempts should not be made to turn their interests outwards to the community. For them, hospital life is only a passing phase.

White, Miller and Polansky,[1] writing from the Austen Riggs Sanitarium, Massachusetts, have summed up the social needs of patients in the concepts of 'sanctuary' and 'social demand'. When a patient is first admitted to hospital, he seeks a place of sanctuary. By a dynamic social process, demand is gradually reimposed until he is ready to return to the community. This process could be reflected in group discussions without raising too many anxieties. Patients are often ready to discuss such matters as why there still exists a stigma against mental illness in some quarters; whether they are likely to encounter this on discharge, and how to respond; what the prospects of employment are; whether to move to another district and 'make a fresh start' after discharge; and other down-to-earth questions of this kind. It might be better in some circumstances to encourage them to do so, rather than fostering discussions about hospital matters, such as food or entertainments, which are of only passing interest to them.

8. *Are high-cost hospitals more efficient than low-cost hospitals?* It is impossible to give a generalized answer to this question, because it depends on how the money is spent. To spend money on more qualified and competent staff, medical equipment, and necessary facilities for patient activities will increase efficiency. To spend it on maintaining outdated and unsatisfactory buildings or on unnecessary elaborations will not.

A better way to frame this question is to ask 'Could most mental hospitals in this country operate more efficiently if they were given more money and more freedom in spending it?' The answer is probably 'Yes'. The special features making for a

[1] R. B. White, S. C. Miller and N. A. Polansky, 'Sanctuary versus Social Demand: the Dilemma of the Therapeutic Community'. Presented to the American Psychiatric Association, May 1955 (unpublished).

lower cost per case in Crown Lodge could be duplicated within the Health Service. We have no grounds for believing that energy, enthusiasm and a desire to preserve the individuality of the patient are a monopoly of private enterprise, or that medical and nursing staff-ratios could not be increased by means of better training facilities, higher salaries, and better working conditions.

9. *Are small hospitals more efficient than large hospitals?* It has been pointed out in Chapter V and elsewhere that large hospitals have certain economic and administrative advantages. A psychiatric unit attached to a general hospital, or a small mental hospital in a mixed group, may have some difficulty in obtaining the staff and equipment which it needs, and in preserving its identity and patterns of administration.

The disadvantages of the large hospital lie in its innate rigidity of organization, the difficulties of communication, and the depersonalizing effect upon patients. Here the small hospital, as a primary social group, has a great advantage.

The ideal would surely be a pattern which combined the advantages of both with the disadvantages of neither. This might be achieved by the creation of small semi-autonomous units loosely associated for financial and administrative purposes—that is, by four or five small hospitals in a separate 'mental group'. Mental deficiency hospitals might also be included in such groups, but we consider that integration of the general medical and psychiatric services is better avoided at group and hospital level.

In most areas, limitations of existing buildings and their geographical location make it difficult to organize groups of this kind at present; but this would be a realistic aim for the future.

10. *Should long-stay and short-stay patients be treated in separate hospitals?* The Ministry of Health's Annual Report for 1959 proposes the setting-up of three types of unit in the future—short-stay, medium-stay and long-stay. If these units are administratively separated from each other, staff may be confined to one type of unit only, with a consequent limitation of experience. Almost inevitably, the long-stay units would get the poorest staff. The prestige-value of this type of work is low, and though there are some doctors and nurses with a vocation to it, they are few in numbers.

The creation of 'mental groups' or psychiatric groups, as suggested above, would overcome this difficulty. Nursing staff would be transferable within the group, so that all types of experience were available, and work with one kind of patient could provide relief from the particular tensions of work with another. Senior medical staff would be responsible for beds in each type of unit. Junior medical staff might be attached to one type only, but serve in each type in turn.

In these circumstances, transfer from a short-stay unit to a medium-stay unit, or from a medium-stay unit to a long-stay unit, would not have about it an air of utter finality and strangeness for the patient. He would still be within the same organization, and he would be treated by people he already knew.

The National Health Service has been in operation for more than half a generation. Now is the time to review its bold experiments, and to experiment again. Given a suitable administrative framework and a reasonable share in available resources, the mental hospital can still be a valuable tool in the hands of the community.

APPENDIX I

METHODOLOGY

SINCE very little work has so far been carried out in England on the administrative and financial aspects of mental hospital life, notes on the methodology used in this survey are given here, in the hope that they may be of use to other research workers, who may be able to refine the methods used and to make improvements on them.

Though the material obtained has been presented here in a different form, to preserve the outlines of the argument, it was actually collected in three separate studies:

(i) What was loosely termed 'the administrative study'. This involved work within the three hospitals: interviews, ward observation, sitting-in at meetings, and the study of records and other data.

(ii) The costing study. This involved the analysis of the hospitals' annual costing returns, time-sheets, salary-sheets, and returns from pharmacists.

(iii) The follow-up study. This involved interview and correspondence with doctors, social workers, and others having professional contact with patients after their discharge.

1. *The Administrative Study*

It was not possible to assess the work of each hospital until we knew the nature of the group of people they were organized to serve. The patient-census was therefore carried out first. This involved working in the Records Office of each hospital in turn, and provided a useful introduction to the hospitals. It was found that in each hospital the Records Office was a focal point in the hospital's life. It was possible to read case-histories, to discuss the progress of individual patients, and to find out a good deal indirectly about the way in which the hospital was organized, and the relationships between groups and individuals. This information was of great value at a later stage, and provided a starting-point for further investigations.

In the two small hospitals, the patient-census covered every patient. It was simply a matter of going through the records and listing the information required, and then putting it on punch-cards.

At Moordale, it was a comparatively simple matter to go through the admission cards of patients, and to take the information from these. At Crown Lodge, there was no comparable system, and it was necessary to go through the patients' case-files, and the admission and discharge books, which of course took a considerably longer time. At Northtown, it was felt that, in the limited time available to us, it was not possible to make a complete census of the 2,750 patients, and so a random sample was taken—one case in five. This means that the patient-census figures for Northtown have not the same degree of accuracy as those for the other two hospitals; but it was already apparent that the difference in patient-structure between Northtown and the other two hospitals was so great that this would not affect the main picture.

The method of assessing social class needs a special note. This is a difficult matter—as John Madge points out, 'No method is free from practical defects and some theoretical naïveté'.[1] It was felt that the Registrar-General's revised classification—the classification usually used for surveys of this kind—was not suitable for the following reasons:

(*a*) The criterion for this classification refers to a standard of social prestige. It has no direct relation either to monetary returns for work as is often supposed, or to the degree of responsibility involved in the work. In this survey, we wished to find out how patients' previous occupations related to the degree of responsibility given to them in hospital, particularly to their participation in decision-making groups; and so the degree of responsibility involved in work was a better criterion.

(*b*) Because the Registrar-General's scheme is based on occupation-groups, it has no grading for people who are 'not gainfully occupied'—students, the unemployed, and people of private means. The census at Crown Lodge, which was the first undertaken, soon showed that a fairly high proportion of the hospital's patients fell into this last group, and that to ignore them would be to falsify the returns. Some patients in all three hospitals have never been gainfully occupied, since their illness has affected them since the time they left school. Others, schizophrenics for example, are sometimes found in work which is clearly unsuited to their social background and education—for instance, a clergyman's son with a university education, who, forced through mental illness to abandon his university course, had eventually become a manual labourer.

In classifying mental patients, there are so many instances of this kind that one cannot ignore them; and there are many patients for whom one feels the only logical classification is 'mental patient'.

[1] *The Tools of Social Science*, 1953.

For long-stay patients who have been in hospital for some years, this is almost a separate category.

We therefore decided to use a simpler form of classification based primarily on the degree of responsibility involved in work. Where the patient was 'not gainfully occupied', we read the case-history, and assigned the patient to a class on the basis of family background and education. Children under working age followed the occupation of father or guardian, non-working wives and widows the occupation of the husband. People of sufficient private means to pay for private treatment were assumed to be 'Class I' if there was no other indication. The three classes were as follows:

Class I: the professions and managerial posts. e.g. doctor, solicitor, accountant, company director, higher civil servant.

Class II: persons engaged on work with some degree of responsibility, but not responsible for policy-making. e.g. primary school teacher, book-keeper, small shopkeeper, executive grade civil servant, foreman.

Class III: persons engaged on work with no degree of responsibility—routine non-manual work and manual work, both skilled and unskilled. e.g. filing clerk, railway porter, dock labourer.

Like all forms of classification, this one is sometimes arbitrary; but its flexible nature made it possible to distinguish between forms of occupation which are covered by the same term but have very different degrees of responsibility. For instance 'engineer' may mean a man who directs the building of a bridge or the man who tightens the nuts and bolts. 'Secretary' may refer to a high-level executive in a major corporation or a shorthand typist. There were of course a number of border-line cases, and here again family backgrounds and education were taken into account.

When the patient-census was complete, we already had some idea of the pattern of relationships within the hospital, and the second part of the administrative survey involved a variety of work using the information already gained as a guide. The administrative study owes much to two previous pieces of research—the method used by T. E. Chester *et al.* in the Acton Society Trust pamphlets 'Hospitals and the State', which involved a similar multi-dimensional approach to an understanding of administrative problems, and the method of Stanton and Schwarz outlined in 'The Mental Hospital', which involved the observation of patterns of relationship and a following-through of administrative processes at ward-level—the level at which they most directly affect the patient.

The research involved spending a period in each hospital in turn, with very few preconceived ideas as to what was being sought for.

It was important to gain an impression of the life of each hospital, the forms which it took, and the problems which emerged in practice. This is a difficult method of research, because one is studying a dynamic situation. One cannot halt the process at any point, and say 'That is what the hospital is like'. Allowance has also to be made for the impact of the research worker on the total situation—an impact which appears to be greater, as one would expect, in a small hospital than in a big one.

Change goes on all the time. Members of staff come and go, patients are admitted and discharged; and it is necessary that the period of observation should be long enough to enable the effect of such changes to be assessed. The short intensive period of observation at each hospital was therefore only a prelude to a period of about a year in which contact was maintained, visits made, and changes noted.

Because the multi-dimensional method was used, the staff had some difficulty in understanding what was being done. There was no simple aim which could be clearly stated in a sentence to those who knew nothing of the methods of social research. A number expected a purely quantitative approach, and asked 'Where's your slide-rule?'

Everybody in a hospital has a clearly-defined role, and nobody has time to waste. There is a clear role-expectation for a doctor, a nurse, a patient, or a lay administrator (though, as we have seen, these expectations are often highly stereotyped, and are not always acceptable to the person concerned). Nobody was quite clear how to treat persons who did not fit into any of these categories, whose progress appeared to be aimless, and in some ways time-wasting.

In each hospital, the medical superintendent was asked for his advice on the question of an approach to the staff and patients, and their replies were very different from one another.

At Crown Lodge, the medical superintendent decided that the best method was for the purpose of the project to be explained at each of the patient-meetings and staff-meetings in turn, in order to allay any possible tensions and anxieties. The staff, as a result, were highly co-operative, and so were short-stay patients, many of whom took a lively interest in the survey; but it was significant that, on the long-stay side of the hospital, where patients were less able to benefit from meetings and discussions, the purpose of the investigation was partially misunderstood, and a rumour went round to the effect that the real purpose was to assess patients' cases, and to make recommendations for discharge—a rather pathetic instance of wishful thinking.

At Moordale, the medical superintendent decided that the purposes of the survey should be explained fully to the medical staff, and this was done; but no general explanation was made to nursing staff or patients. Individual explanations were made where these seemed advisable.

At both Crown Lodge and Moordale, there was a sense of being assimilated to the hospital's pattern—of being drawn into a tight in-group, and of having to make responses to it. In a small primary social group—particularly one which is psychodynamically orientated—formal role-playing is not enough. It was necessary to make contacts on a deeper and more personal basis, and we were soon regarded as 'part of the team'.

At Northtown, no explanations were necessary. The hospital had been the subject of several earlier social surveys by another university, and was used to 'university people' and their special approach to hospital life. The role was a much simpler one. The staff were friendly and co-operative; but relationships were more formal. A research worker was an outsider with a special job to do, and personal relationships did not develop outside that role. In a sense this made the work easier, because there was never a danger of losing an objective approach—a factor which had constantly to be kept in mind in the two smaller hospitals.

Reference has already been made to the difficulty of being apparently aimless in a society which is busy and has definite purposes; and it was found necessary on the wards to have some apparent purpose. Simply to sit down in a ward and to observe what was going on would be enough to make the whole process of ward administration and ward relationships highly self-conscious and highly atypical. We therefore adopted a practice well known to those who wish to avoid the sergeant-major's eye in the Army—such apparently purposeful occupations as counting the windows, measuring the wards, drawing plans—which were enough to give an appearance of occupation until conversation developed. Meanwhile, the normal routine of the ward went on undisturbed.

Sitting-in at meetings was easier. It was possible to sit in the back row, and to make unobtrusive notes. Where small groups of patients were interviewed, this was done with the advice of the doctor, but without the presence of any member of staff. This provided some difficulty in that it was necessary to lead the group—or at least to keep it talking on the right lines—and at the same time to keep a verbatim record of conversations. The use of a tape-recorder was rejected on the grounds that it might alter the content of conversation. People who are not used to tape-recording are often self-conscious, and they might well have felt that tape-recorded material was not confidential, since it could be played back to the staff. The idea of a concealed tape-recorder, or a concealed shorthand writer, was rejected on ethical grounds. It is scarcely fair to ask people to talk freely and in confidence if such methods are used. So it was necessary to make quick, brief notes with some word of excuse and then to type them up immediately the session was over, while the whole course of conversation and the personalities of those who took part were still fresh in mind, and before any rationalization could affect the content. The conversations quoted were recorded in this manner.

Interviewing psychiatrists had its own difficulties. Psychiatrists are used to interviewing other people, and are apt, when interviewed themselves, to be far more interested in the techniques of the interview than in its subject-matter. At first, an attempt was made to carry out unconstructed interviews—the aim being to find out what the psychiatrists themselves thought were the priorities for discussion. Long silences sometimes led to irritability, and once or twice to momentary hostility—'If you don't know what you want to ask, why have you come here at all?' Such responses—very similar to those they themselves obtained from individual patients or from groups by the use of the same technique—led eventually to useful conversations; but it was felt that better results were obtained on the whole from purely informal contacts. Where this was not possible, psychiatrists were approached with a number of definite questions which could be answered, in the hope that, when they had been answered, the interview would develop along freer and less formalized lines.

Participant research in a dynamic situation has complications. As one psychiatrist said, 'When I deal with people professionally, they lie on a couch, and I sit out of sight and say very little. You have to be in the situation—taking part in it with an appearance of spontaneity, yet being objective about it at the same time.' This double approach—involvement and non-involvement—meant that attitudes and responses to specific situations had to be thought out fairly carefully; and that a fairly sharp distinction had to be made between information which could be used for the project, and information given in personal confidence. Information given 'off the record' has not been used directly in this report, though it often contributed a good deal to a general understanding of problems. Facts about one hospital—unless they were matters of general knowledge—were not mentioned in conversations at the other two. This rule held good even in relation to our psychiatric adviser, who was on the staff of one of the three hospitals; and with his consent.

In interviews, neither staff nor patients were pressed to say more than they wished to say on a particular subject, and they were always given an assurance that confidences would be respected both in and out of the hospital. Material given in interviews was cross-checked wherever possible—sometimes several times over.

The initial periods of observation at the three hospitals were completed from June to November 1958. Notes on each hospital were typed and filed day by day during this period, so that there were three fairly large dossiers by November. There were two main ways in which this material might have been subject to bias: first by over-involvement and a lack of objectivity—though this factor had been constantly kept in mind; and second, by the nature of the role which we had fulfilled. In each hospital, although there was some confusion as to the exact role, we were accepted as being of 'doctor-status'. This gave many advantages, and it would have been difficult to study the administration of the hospital at all levels from a lower status-position. At the same time, it involved some limitations on the material collected, particularly where the nursing staff were concerned. The way in which a nurse speaks of her work to a 'doctor' may not be at all similar to the way in which she would speak of it to another nurse; and the routine which goes on in the ward when a 'doctor' is present may be quite different from what happens when the nursing staff and the patients are alone.

To check on these factors, five student volunteers were sent to the hospitals during university vacations, to work as assistant nurses, and to make their own reports on what they experienced. They went with the full consent and understanding of the medical superintendent and matron in each case; but so far as other nursing staff were concerned, they were simply students acting as relief nurses in a busy period. A number of mental hospitals which are short-staffed take on students for short periods in this way during vacations. They wore uniform, lived in the nurses' home, and received the usual rate of pay for an assistant nurse, carrying out the normal duties under the authority of the nursing staff.

They were given no definite briefing as to the kind of report which was expected from them, since it was felt that a specific approach would prejudice the nature of their observations. All five produced long and interesting reports. These confirmed the impressions gained in the previous summer's period of research, and did not reveal the existence of any noticeable bias in the material already collected. They provided some interesting sidelights on the attitude of the nursing staff to their work, and extracts from three reports are given in Appendix II.

2. *The Costing Study*

The cost analysis involved the use of more direct methods. Expenditure accounting is efficiently done in all three hospitals, but classification of expense is in each case on a basis of broad subjective headings only.

The initial task was to arrange for the expenditure during a suitable period of time to be analysed on a common basis in all three hospitals. Both Moordale and Northtown employ the Ministry of Health's modified costing scheme, and because the heads of expense specified in that scheme were already costed at those hospitals, we decided to adopt them for the purposes of the survey. Crown Lodge, as an independent hospital, does not account under the Ministry's scheme, but employs an analysis of expenditure appropriate to its special purposes. It was thus necessary for all the expenditure at Crown Lodge during the selected accounting period to be re-analysed under the heads provided in the Ministry's scheme, in common form with the figures already available at Moordale and Northtown. This proved to be a considerable task, only possible because of the willing co-operation we received from the secretary and his staff at Crown Lodge.

The figures provided by this initial analysis are presented in Table 23 in the main text. They are total expenditure and average cost per patient-week in the three hospitals during an accounting year ending during the year ended 31st March 1958.

As has been explained in the main text this initial analysis did little more than provide illustrations in financial terms of historical, physical and organizational differences between the three hospitals.

In the second stage of the cost analysis an attempt was made to divide the total expenditure of the hospitals under certain heads between long-stay and the short-stay patients, so as to provide average costs per week and per case for each category. Enquiry at this stage was concentrated on expenditure under three heads; the costs of medical care, nursing care, and drugs and dressings, for several reasons. In the first instance, both salaries costs and stores issues are capable of analysis by well-tried and reasonably accurate accounting methods. To have extended the field of the enquiry to cover other factors, for example repairs and maintenance costs, would have involved the introduction of more or less arbitrary methods of expense apportionment. Secondly, the costed expenses are those which contribute most directly to the patient's recovery. Environmental factors are, of course, important, but their effect is indirect and not easily capable of expression in terms of cost. Thirdly, the whole of the work of the second costing stage was necessarily undertaken by the research workers. Costing in the Hospitals Service generally suffers from lack of sufficient adequately trained staff, and this is particularly true of mental hospitals, which have less experience of costing than have most general hospitals.

The amount of time available for detailed analysis of costs limited the range of the enquiry.

In order to determine the cost of medical care, doctors in all three hospitals were asked to complete records of their employment. Simple forms were issued, providing separate spaces for each half-hour of the day and each hour of the night, in which the doctors were asked to indicate by symbols the kinds of work on which they had been engaged.

The symbols were:

A—clinical care of short-stay patients.
B—clinical care of long-stay patients.
Z—administration.
M—meetings or consultations with colleagues.
O—miscellaneous.
X—on call.

Only time spent in the hospital was recorded on the forms. Records of extra-mural activities of medical staff were obtained from the medical superintendents of the hospitals.

Each doctor was allocated a code-symbol, and this symbol, and not his name, appeared on the forms issued to him. Four forms were issued to each doctor, one for each week costed, together with four addressed envelopes for the direct despatch of the completed records to the University. This rather complicated procedure ensured confidentiality, and prevented those taking part from making comparisons which might have led to the submission of returns recording some conception of the ideal, rather than the actual expenditure of time.

Filling in these forms was a task of some magnitude. It involved an effort of memory on the part of the doctors, and took some time. Nevertheless, the medical staff were most conscientious in completing the records, often telephoning for advice on the classification of a particular activity, and a reasonable degree of standardization of analysis resulted.

From the doctors' returns it was possible to discover the pattern of employment of each during the test month. Each doctor's salary, at the rate applicable during the test month, was then apportioned among the various categories of his employment in proportion to the amounts of time spent. Due allowance was, of course, made for extra-mural activities.

By adding together the individual doctors' figures, it was then possible to discover what part of the total medical salaries cost of each hospital in the test month was applicable to each of the categories of activity for which records had been kept. These figures were effectively a sample of the allocation of doctors' time weighted for relative levels of remuneration.

The sample figures were then used to divide the total cost of medical salaries during the costed year to 31st March 1958 between the activity categories. The costs allocated by this method to clinical care of short-stay and long-stay patients were then applied in the following formula to give separate costs of medical care per patient-week for each class of patient:

$$\begin{array}{l}\text{Proportion of total expenditure}\\ \text{on (e.g.) medical salaries in re-}\\ \text{spect of short-stay patients in}\\ \text{(e.g.) Crown Lodge (calculated}\\ \text{as described above)}\end{array} \times \frac{7}{365} \times \frac{1}{\begin{array}{c}\text{Number of short-stay}\\ \text{patients in Crown Lodge}\end{array}}$$

A similar costing method was employed in calculating the cost of nursing care for each class of patient. Lists of nurses on each ward day-by-day over a four-week period were supplied by matrons and chief male nurses. Nurses who moved from one ward to another during the course of a day were traced. Many nurses were engaged continuously in the care of one class or other of the patients, and their salaries were allocated directly to the class concerned. Others, whose work was more varied, were costed in like manner to the doctors.

The enquiry provided analyses of time from which it proved possible to divide the total nursing salaries paid at each hospital in the test month between clinical care of short-stay patients, clinical care of long-stay patients, and other duties. The sample figures thus calculated were applied to total nursing salaries costs in the year to 31st March 1958 in the manner described for doctors' salaries.

The pharmacist at each hospital was asked to keep detailed records of drugs and dressings supplied to each class of patients during the test month. These records, when costed up at prices ruling during the test month, provided a sample for application to the total drugs and dressings cost in year ended 31st March 1958 in the manner described.

Average patient-week costs for the two classes of patients calculated in the manner described are presented in the main text in Tables 25–27. The average patient-week costs for short-stay patients are shown alternatively as average costs per case in Table 29. Average costs per case have been calculated by the following formula:

$$\text{Average cost per patient-week} \times \frac{\begin{array}{c}\text{Average length of stay of}\\ \text{first admissions}\end{array}}{7}$$

The test period for the construction of the samples of cost of medical and nursing care and drugs and dressings was in each case 28 days, but not the same 28 days was used at each hospital. Local difficulties—changes in medical staff, abnormal amounts of sickness among nurses, staff holidays, etc.—produce atypical situations. For this reason we decided to allow the hospitals to select that period of 28 days during three months which was considered to present the most typical picture of their activities. Since the period chosen was to be regarded as typical of a whole year, it was considered more important to have the samples representative than to have them coincident in time.

3. *The Follow-up Study*

The original plan was to match groups of 100 or more patients from each of the three hospitals for follow-up—matching on the criteria of sex, age, diagnosis and occupation.

Selection of cases was begun, matching age and sex; but it was found difficult to match occupations, even in the three simple groups used for the patient-census. After two months' work, we discovered that it would be necessary, in order to get three matched groups of 100 patients each, to go back to patients discharged early in 1953. This was felt to be useless—not only would patients who had been out of hospital for over six years be difficult to trace, but those discharged before 1955 would not have been treated with the new drugs which came into use then. These drugs have in some cases altered the prognosis considerably, and there is no value in mixing in one group patients discharged before and after 1955 for this reason.

Although matching had been achieved in some cases, it was a purely notional matching. If somebody was described as a 'company director' in Crown Lodge, he was not necessarily the same kind of company director as might be found in Northtown. It was often necessary to stretch the categories considerably in order to make people fit.

In view of these considerations, the attempt to match large groups was abandoned, and an unmatched sample from each hospital was taken. This consisted of patients discharged at least two years before the follow-up study, since the medical superintendents agreed that the greatest probability of relapse occurred within a period of two years from the date of discharge. This meant that, if patients were to relapse, that relapse would probably have taken place by the time enquiries were made. Since unmatched samples were taken, it was possible to complete the samples with people who had been discharged within six months of one another, thus getting more homogeneous groups. Patients were selected simply in order of discharge, running backwards from a date two years before the date of selection. Multiple admissions were excluded, since we could obtain a more controlled situation by testing the effect of one period of treatment at the hospital taking part in the survey. All the patients in the sample are therefore first admissions. Patients suffering from illness of known organic origin (such as the psychoses of old age) were also excluded, because the prognosis is poorer in many such cases.

In this way, a sample was obtained which gave a fairly typical picture of discharge from each hospital, but of course the samples were not comparable. In order that we might have some comparable data, cards in these three samples were then matched where possible for age, sex, occupation and diagnosis; 30 cards from each hospital were found to match, and these form the basis of the small matched sample discussed on pages 149 to 151.

Letters and forms were drawn up for despatch to local authorities and general practitioners. These asked for information in confidence on a top sheet which bore the patient's name and address, and his code number for the investigation. Only the form, which bore merely the code number, was to be returned. Each form was accompanied by a stamped addressed envelope, and was designed so that it could be filled in very quickly by a series of ticks and crosses.

The method adopted at Crown Lodge was to contact general practitioners first, since it is not usual for referrals to be made to local authorities from this hospital. When these methods failed, the medical superintendent took the personal responsibility of finding out from general practitioners or relatives what had happened to the patient.

At Moordale and Northtown, the method adopted was to contact local authorities first, since all cases are referred to the local authority of the area to which the patient is discharged unless the patient specifically requests that this should not be done. The material obtained from local authorities was very patchy in character. Some local authorities were prepared to ask their workers to make a special visit if the case was unknown to them. Others, through apathy or a genuine shortage of staff, returned most forms marked 'No information'.

We should hesitate to judge the efficiency of a local authority Mental Health Service by the amount of information it was able to supply. Some excellent case-workers are poor record-keepers; and the inability to supply information from files may reflect a lack of clerical assistance rather than a poor case-work service.

When the local authority failed to supply full information, a form was sent to the patient's general practitioner. Here again, the response was uneven. Some were extremely helpful; others seem to have regarded this as just one more irritating item in a large morning mail, and to have consigned both the original request and the tactful reminder sent six weeks later direct to the waste-paper basket. Again, this may have reflected overwork and lack of secretarial help rather than lack of good-will.

At this point, it was necessary to find other sources of information. Some of the patients were traced by informal contacts which they had maintained with members of the hospital staff. This was possible in a number of cases at Moordale, where the hospital keeps informal notes of what has happened to patients in their case-files, and where, since the area is a rural one, information is more easily come by. One patient was traced by means of a newspaper cutting which had been clipped from a local newspaper and sent to the Records Office by a nurse.

At Northtown, by contrast, the official channels of after-care were highly efficient, but there was very little informal contact.

These methods provided over 90 per cent of replies in each case; but there remained a hard core in which the patient had moved, changed his general practitioner, or refused after-care of any kind. The records of other mental hospitals in the area and of out-patient clinics were searched. Sometimes we obtained a little information which led on to another source—the warden of a hostel, a probation officer, or an almoner. Every possible source was tried apart from a direct visit to the patient. This was partly because information obtained directly from patients might be unreliable in some cases; but the main reason was that we felt it undesirable to visit patients for a purpose unconnected with their own welfare. Patients have a right to privacy. This is not invaded by a request for confidential information from a doctor or worker, provided that the information is coded on punch-cards, and not kept in a form which might be understood by someone outside the research team; but we felt that privacy would be invaded, and distress might be caused, if we approached patients personally. A visit two years or more after leaving hospital would bring the period of acute illness vividly back to mind. Confidence might be broken, since a relative or a neighbour might overhear details which had been kept from them by the patient. There was a risk that a visit might cause distress or annoyance to a patient sufficient to cause a relapse; and we felt that we had no right to visit patients for a non-therapeutic and possibly anti-therapeutic purpose.

The indirect method of approach produced a response of 97 per cent (Crown Lodge), 98 per cent (Northtown) and 97·7 per cent (Moordale), which was greater than we had anticipated.

Personal visits for follow-up enquiry purposes are in our opinion justified only if the follow-up is made by a psychiatrist or social worker who already has a rapport with the patient. This of necessity restricts their use to small groups. They cannot be used effectively for comparative purposes, since this would involve several psychiatrists and social workers with different standards, each following up his own patients. They cannot be used for large-scale studies, since visiting is very time-consuming, and the whole process of follow-up must be completed in a few weeks if the first results are to be comparable with the last ones; and they must be restricted to those patients who have remained near the hospital because of travelling difficulties—a fact which may considerably bias the sample.

Where large groups and patients treated by different psychiatrists are involved, the postal survey is preferable, with two qualifications: questions must be capable of an objective answer (e.g. 'Is the patient now in normal employment?') rather than matters of opinion (e.g. 'Has the patient recovered?'). Unless questions are confined to matters of ascertainable fact, answers will obviously represent widely divergent standards. Second, there should be a previous link between the person requesting information and the person who is asked to provide it. In most cases, we visited medical officers of health, and telephoned or wrote a preliminary letter to general practitioners if they were not already known to us. This undoubtedly contributed greatly to the high percentage of responses obtained; and the few failures were all in cases where we had been unable to trace the doctors or local authority responsible.

APPENDIX II

STUDENTS' REPORTS

Crown Lodge

My first impression of the hospital consisted of thick carpets and arrays of brightly coloured chrysanthemums along all the corridors which were wide and airy, with large windows overlooking the green grounds. No bars, no locked doors and, at first glance, very little supervision of any kind. . . . The Treatment Ward was divided into two: one half was in a hospital ward where the patients were often not allowed to dress, the second consisting of dormitories and single rooms along the corridor whose occupants used the dining-room, drawing-room and television room downstairs. . . .

The only locked door, even on the ward, where several of the patients were suicidal, was to the ward duty room where all the drugs were kept. I found the greatest strain of nursing was not looking after the patients physically but keeping careful watch on them all without making such vigilance apparent. Several of the patients were given to wandering and it needed great tact to coax them back into the vicinity of the ward. Despite the increased responsibility engendered by the unlocked door, the nurses preferred the free atmosphere which they said helped them to get to know the patients as friends and not jailers. Emphasis was laid on remaining in one ward so that the bond between individual nurses and patients could be strengthened, and the nurses complained bitterly if they were moved to a strange ward. . . . Another factor which helped to create not only a free but friendly atmosphere was the use of Christian names both by the patients and by the nurses amongst themselves. Even the sister used her Christian name, but I must admit that I often popped 'sister' in front as, at first, it seemed quite disrespectful for me to use her Christian name alone. All these small details added up to the role of the nurse as friend and companion rather than as warder in a purely official capacity. . . .

Discipline at Crown Lodge was automatically laxer than in a normal general hospital from the very organization of the place, emphasizing friendship between staff as well as between patients and staff. . . .

It was interesting to note how the patients reacted to my introduction into the ward and from this I could gauge, to a large extent, how they felt towards the nursing staff. . . . A few of them suffered from a severe persecution complex as far as the nursing staff were concerned and would come to me with their requests as though I was an ally among a hostile group. . . . Some patients are always asking interminable questions and demanding all kinds of permission and privileges which are all beyond the nurse's ability to grant. The stock answer to such a statement as 'I'm not going to have the treatment (E.C.T.) tomorrow', must inevitably be 'You'll have to see the doctor about that'. Obviously this type of answer is evasive but the ordinary nurse has no alternative; she has a routine to get through and has no power over such matters in any case. . . . On the whole the relationship between staff and patients was relaxed and trusting. The patients seemed to be satisfied with the treatment accorded them; they were allowed their most personal possessions and usually a fixed amount of pocket money which could be spent on a variety of things at the canteen, provided they were allowed downstairs. All their property was carefully marked and hung in wardrobes or placed in particular drawers near the ward. Indeed, as much as possible was done to preserve the individual's feeling of independence and familiarity, which is very important.

One drawback the nurses voiced in trying to establish concrete relationships with the patients was inherent in the fact that Crown Lodge was a private hospital. The patients were paying for service and the people who had to do the serving were the nurses themselves. In most hospitals, even the ordinary nurse carries a certain aura of authority but here the atmosphere was more one of master-servant than of patient-nurse. Some of the nurses definitely disliked this particular aspect of their work which to them was personified in the fact that they had to serve the patients at table. In fact, one nurse made the charge against the hospital that it was too much like an hotel and not enough like a hospital. He intimated that this state of affairs affected the efficiency of treatment to a certain extent. . . . Only having a brief experience of Crown Lodge I cannot personally subscribe to this view. . . .

The Mixed Unit is a new experimental unit designed to accustom the sexes to mixing again after long terms of segregation, before going home. Its success cannot be judged as yet, but the nurses say that the old gentlemen, as old they usually are, hold aloof from the ladies although there are one or two devoted couples to prove the exception. One old gentleman from this unit who does the garden is continually dogged by one persistent lady, who never leaves his side whatever the weather. Even if this unit does not renew companionship between the sexes it at least revives the normal antagonism, which is a healthy sign. . . .

Working at Crown Lodge was an experience I shall always value. . . . Working with these people, getting to know and understand them, has made me realize that mental illness is not a subject remote from me personally but a reality which someday I might come up against myself. In these people I could see exaggerated images not only of myself but of people I know, my mother, for instance, with her acute excitability. Learning how to deal with the mentally sick will help me to understand people I meet every day.

Northtown

Since this is to be a personal and not an objective account of my experience, I think it will help if I give a brief outline of the attitude of mind in which I approached this work. This is important because it affected the way in which I noticed things. I tried very hard not to have any preconceptions of what this work would be like but, inevitably, I had at the back of my mind certain ideas and expectations about the patients and about the hospital. I expected violent patients and a depressing hospital atmosphere—ideas picked up from plays and secondhand accounts of life in a mental hospital. The last thing I expected was that I would enjoy working there.

I arrived at the gates of Northtown Hospital on a dreary December morning. A new patient and his father arrived at the same time and we walked up the drive together. I felt rather nervous and apprehensive about the new environment and people I was coming to and I tried to understand what a new patient would feel like. I was used to moving about from one group of people to another. It would be much more difficult for this young boy to get used to his new friends and surroundings and I wondered how the hospital would tackle the problem of helping him to settle in.

My first impression of the buildings was one of vastness and ugliness. However, once inside, we found brightly decorated corridors with pictures and a large number of potted plants.

The friendliness and welcome of the matron and other members of the staff was also a pleasant surprise, since I had expected to be overawed by the dignity traditionally attached to hospital hierarchy. . . .

The biggest surprise came when I first went on duty later in the same day. Just before the deputy matron took me on to the ward she warned me that I might be rather shocked since I had never met mentally ill people before. This made me feel even more apprehensive than I had felt before. . . .

The patients were friendly, co-operative and generally well-behaved. I had expected violences, excitement, detachment or evident strangeness but I found very little of these things. My surprise was even greater when I found that I was able to carry on normal conversation with patients. . . .

The whole atmosphere of the ward impressed me for its bright friendliness. I tried to take into account the fact that this was Christmastime and that many preparations were being made for the holiday, but I felt that this prevailing mood of cheerfulness could not have been 'got up' for Christmas unless it genuinely existed.

The reason why I have dealt so fully with these first impressions is that they completely changed the attitude with which I approached the job. I said in the first paragraph that my preconceptions coloured the way in which I observed what I saw in the hospital. They did this in an indirect, rather dialectical way: the thesis—preconceptions expecting the worst; the antithesis—first impressions so favourable that, for a while, I saw everything in a similar light; the synthesis—an attempt to observe objectively. . . .

Christmas decorations: The theme of these on this ward was to be an English flower garden and our job today was to twist narrow strips of yellow paper for laburnum. This was very simple and suitable for the patients to help with. I was rather surprised to notice that the staff waited for patients to volunteer to help instead of inviting their help. I also noticed that many of the patients needed constant assistance and encouragement. Even a simple task like this was extremely difficult for some but they did respond to any help that was given. However, most of the staff did not seem to bother with encouraging the patients who were helping; they seemed to be more concerned with the task itself and were eager to get the decorations finished. I felt in this way they were missing a valuable opportunity of helping the patient to enjoy working with a group and play some part in the life of the ward. However, when I tried to help some of these patients who were finding the job a little difficult, I could quite understand the nurses' reluctance. It needed great patience and perseverance. It was easy for me; I was fresh to the job and had not been working so hard as the others on the domestic work of the ward. But, since the patients so enjoyed joining in with this simple job and appreciated any help and encouragement so much, I was very disappointed that this did not seem to be an accepted part of the nurse's job.

The staff were kind and considerate to all the patients, although sometimes, if a patient behaved awkwardly, they would change this attitude rather as a mother keeps a stern face when her child has done something wrong. In fact, the misbehaving patient was normally treated like a naughty child. For example, Ellen, a young girl of about seventeen, had been rather noisy all morning. She offered to help with the decorations. One of the nurses was called away to the telephone. As she went, she turned and said to me in a loud voice, 'Don't let that Ellen touch the scissors.' Ellen was offended and humiliated and I felt that the nurse could have told me in a quieter and more tactful way instead of letting both Ellen and everybody else know that we did not trust her. . . .

When I arrived, the deputy matron took charge of me, showed me to my room, helped me into my uniform and insisted on lending me crockery and giving me some food. I very soon felt at home. The welcome given to patients was rather different. A nurse from the admissions ward met them in the main office and brought them up to the ward. There they were bathed immediately, dressed in night-gowns and dressing-gowns and brought into the day-room for tea with their wet hair still tangled and uncombed. They were not properly introduced to the other patients and were put to bed immediately after tea. No wonder that they felt strange and frightened! They were not treated unkindly but I felt that their entrance to the hospital could have been managed more imaginatively and sympathetically. Of course, this would be quite impossible with the present staff-patient ratio.

I was struck by the counting of knives and forks after each meal and in the way in which they were locked up in a large box. It is quite understandable that this is necessary in a large ward where there are a few patients likely to attempt suicide but I disliked the way in which knives and forks were collected from the tables as soon as the patients had finished using them. Surely this could have been left to the end of the meal! . . .

The Insulin Department: The afternoons are free for reading, table tennis, and occupational therapy. . . . Most of the time the nurses sat with the patients reading women's magazines. I had heard the nurses grumbling about the boredom of the afternoons and now I could understand what they meant. As far as they could see, their nursing task finished with the morning's treatment. What opportunities they were missing for making friends with patients, helping them to gain confidence by teaching them new skills in needlework and handwork and encouraging them to mix with the male patients! Here was the only place in the hospital where staff had the time and opportunity to help patients socially and the nurses grumbled because they were bored. I am afraid that I rather stuck my neck out here. I soon became tired of sitting and doing nothing so I suggested a game of table tennis with one of the patients. Nobody seemed interested so I played with one of the male nurses. Then one of our patients jumped up and asked for a game and soon three of them were taking it in turns to play, not very expertly, it is true, but with much enjoyment and laughter. I do not want to criticize the nursing staff in this respect; their approach to the job was full of genuine care and interest. It was simply that they were not expected to carry their nursing role from the physical sphere into the social sphere, and did not seem to understand the important part they could play in helping the patient to live with other people and establish relationships with them.

The Refractory Ward: As its name suggests, this ward is for dangerous and potentially violent patients. It was called by this name in front of the patients, which I thought was a bad thing since it would confirm any ideas they had of being a nuisance. In fact, it makes them sound like naughty children instead of sick people. . . .

Staff relationships here were the most unsatisfactory that I came across in the whole hospital. The sister was very aloof from the rest of the staff and the nurses seemed to approach their work in a rather grudging way. While I was there a Christmas present, a box of sweets, arrived addressed to 'The Staff on Ward ——' One of the nurses remarked to me, 'We'll not see that again.' I do not know if she was right, but it certainly seems to indicate that the atmosphere between the staff was not so healthy here as in the other wards which I saw. . . .

With one exception, all the nurses I have met seem to have the idea at the back of their minds that they must always be doing something and that to sit down and chat with a patient would be 'slacking'. One of the nurses told me about something that had happened while she was working in the Neurosis Unit. She had become really interested in Bet, a young girl of about her own age. They had a great deal in common although Bet had had a most unhappy home background. Mary felt that she was really helping Bet by making friends with her. One day they were sitting, talking in the lounge when the doctor came. Mary jumped up immediately, feeling rather guilty at being discovered like that. But the doctor said, 'Sit down, nurse.' Mary said that the sister would not have been pleased to find her like that. . . .

From my reading there has emerged the fact that the mental hospital can help its patients in two main ways. Firstly, by direct methods of treatment such as electro-convulsant treatment, deep insulin therapy, leucotomy, occupational therapy and psychotherapy. Secondly, by the indirect, but no less effective, method of encouraging the patient to make sound personal and group relationships with staff and fellow patients.

In this second type of treatment, the role of the nurse is a vital one. She is a member of staff who works closest to the patient and therefore has the best opportunities for observing him over long periods and when he is most relaxed. Also, she has the best opportunities for getting to know him, helping him by showing that she sympathizes, trying to understand him and his needs and helping to restore the self-respect which he might have lost when he entered the hospital.

At Northtown I found every facility for the first kind of treatment but little or none of the second kind. I did indeed find therapeutic friendships and group relationships between patients in the convalescent ward and in the Neurosis Unit but I got the impression that the staff had played very little part in encouraging this. . . . In fact, at Northtown, the nurse's role was chiefly that of custodian and domestic help.

All the time there was the sense of pressure to get things done, the bed to be made, meals to be served, always something. One got the impression that the patients were simply fitted into the daily routine instead of that being evolved on the basis of their needs. I have mentioned that patients were often treated like children. If one misbehaved the reproof was almost invariably, 'Oh, you naughty girl!'

What I felt to be lacking was a fundamental attitude of respect towards patients, the idea that they were adult human beings. Perhaps this is why the staff did not enjoy working in the Neurosis Unit, because they had to remember this fact. . . .

Until today, I had felt rather impatient with the nurses because they seemed to be so blind to the social and personal side of their work, neglecting many opportunities for helping patients by talking to them and showing genuine interest in their affairs. However, today I could really sympathize. To talk to a mentally ill person requires great effort, patience and perseverance. Sometimes the conversation appears to be making no effect, or the patient's replies are irrelevant to one's initial remark. When one is kept busy working physically hard the task seems to be twice as difficult, especially if one is pressed for time and knows that there is a job which urgently needs doing. . . .

There are two main reasons why the indirect methods of treatment which I have briefly mentioned are not put into practice there. They are rather obvious. First, there are not enough staff. For such methods to be put effectively into practice there would need to be a higher proportion of staff to patients. . . .

Second, as far as I could gather, the training given to a mental nurse directs very little attention to the importance of her role in the personal and social relationships of the ward. . . .

I have tried to give some idea of the limitations and difficulties with which Northtown Hospital has to contend in its task of healing the mentally ill. Within these limitations I think it is doing its work admirably. Everywhere I went, patients and their relatives were full of praise for what was being done. The atmosphere was definitely not depressing as I had anticipated. . . .

I enjoyed and valued my experience of working there and I hope that I have not been too broad and sweeping in my remarks.

Moordale

In order to take up mental nursing one requires a definite sense of vocation, for not only is the training course long but the work is tiring both physically and mentally, the hours are rather unusual and the pay is not very high. A student nurse living in the nurses' hostel only receives about £10 a month after deductions for board and lodging, taxes, insurance and laundry. Mental nursing is an extremely tiring work. In the chronic wards a nurse may continually be lifting patients who are unable to help themselves—and who don't even wish to be moved. In other wards, because of staff shortages, nurses may have to do the work of two. In addition to this physical strain there is the mental strain of thinking for one's patients and of trying to do one job whilst keeping on the alert lest someone else tries to run away or commit suicide. . . .

There is another difficulty about mental nursing which is important. That is that so often the work seems to be showing no positive result, particularly in the chronic wards—and so often the work fails to be appreciated. Patients, because of their illness, may feel the nurse, whilst doing her best, is really not interested in them or feel that she is being unkind. I never saw a nurse be unkind to a patient but I have several times heard a patient complain of the treatment she received whilst, in actual fact, the nurse was only doing her duty. I can now understand the fantastic stories of wrongful detention in mental homes by former patients! . . .

The nursing assistant is untrained but she can compensate for much of this lack of training by experience and length of stay. Many nursing assistants are middle-aged married women who have been at the hospital for many years. They know their patients well and soon notice any change in a patient's condition. Often they are on much better terms with their patients than the sister, who may not have been there so long and not been in such close contact with them, or the student nurse, whom many of the patients may regard as being too young or immature to understand their problems. . . .

The work of the sister and the part she plays in the life of the ward varies greatly. . . . Some sisters rarely stop to eat a real meal and are continually supervising their staff, whereas others seem to take very little part in the life of the ward and assume that the staff understand their responsibilities. . . .

I think that the relationships between the staff were generally good at Moordale. . . .

The size of the mental hospital is extremely important because too large a unit will make the patient feel lost in a crowd. He may feel an insignificant member, just another number in the case book. . . . Moordale is, perhaps, about the optimum size for a mental hospital. Its 400 beds can be maintained at an economical cost and its patients do not feel lost in a large crowd. A very happy community spirit pervades the hospital. Patients on one ward have close friends on other wards and in the hostel. . . . As there are between 30–40 people on each ward each patient can feel that she is a member of a small group. I think that this feeling of a happy group—which is a very new feeling for many patients since often their illness has been caused by their inability to make relationships with others—is intensified by the light jobs which the patients carry out in the morning. Each patient has his own task to do and so gains a sense of responsibility to himself and to the ward. . . . The hospital is like a village in that everyone knows everyone else and in that each is dependent upon the other. Patients on the way to recovery are only too willing to do small favours for those who are less well, and to try to encourage them to recovery. . . .

The nurse must be happy in her work or else she will not be able to give her full attention to the patient. I liked the atmosphere at Moordale and thought that it was quite a happy place, despite the miseries which some of the patients are undergoing. One day after I had been singing 'Daisy, Daisy' with one of the chronic patients (it's her favourite song) the old lady beamed at me and said, 'We have some good times don't we?' . . .

INDEX

For Product Safety Concerns and Information please contact our EU representative GPSR@taylorandfrancis.com
Taylor & Francis Verlag GmbH, Kaufingerstraße 24, 80331 München, Germany

www.ingramcontent.com/pod-product-compliance
Lightning Source LLC
LaVergne TN
LVHW011129300926
849160LV00008B/575

* 9 7 8 0 4 1 5 8 6 4 1 8 3 *